THE
FOUR
TEMPERAMENTS

THE

FOUR
TEMPERAMENTS

A REDISCOVERY OF THE ANCIENT WAY OF
UNDERSTANDING CHARACTER AND HEALTH

RANDY ROLFE, J.D., M.A.

Illustrations by Robert Rayevsky

MARLOWE & COMPANY
NEW YORK

THE FOUR TEMPERAMENTS:
A Rediscovery of the Ancient Way of Understanding Health and Character

Copyright © Randy Rolfe 2002
Illustrations copyright © Robert Rayevsky 2002
www.rayevsky.com

Published by
Marlowe & Company
An Imprint of Avalon Publishing Group Incorporated
161 William Street, 16th Floor
New York, NY 10038

The information in this book is intended to help readers make informed decisions
about their health and the health of their loved ones. It is not intended to be a
substitute for treatment by or the advice and care of a professional health care
provider. While the author and publisher have endeavored to ensure that the
information presented is accurate and up to date, they are not responsible for
adverse effects or consequences sustained by any person using this book.

Library of Congress Cataloging-in-Publication Data

Rolfe, Randy.
The four temperaments : a rediscovery of the ancient way
of understanding health and character / by Randy Rolfe.
p. cm.
Includes bibliographical references and index.
ISBN 1-56924-562-2
ISBN 978-1-569-24562-0
1. Health—Miscellanea. 2. Four temperaments. 3. Medicine, Ancient.
4. Medicine, Greek and Roman. 5. Self-care, Health—Miscellanea. I. Title.
RA776.5 .R64 2002
613—dc21   2002075111

DESIGNED BY PAULINE NEUWIRTH, NEUWIRTH & ASSOCIATES, INC.

Printed in the United States of America
Distributed by Publishers Group West

To Spirit who connects us all

Contents

List of Figures

Introduction Temperamentally Yours I

Chapter 1 Your Four Humors 15
  A Brief History of Humorology

Chapter 2 What's Your Humor? 25
  The Ancient Masters of the Humors

Chapter 3 Your Humoral Physique: 43
  Physical Traits by the Humors
  The Humors and the Playing Cards

Chapter 4 Your Humoral Temperament: 61
  Personality by the Humors
  The Modern Masters of the Humors

Chapter 5 Your Humoral Relationships: 77
  Romance and Friends by the Humors
  Duality and the Humors
  Vibrational Health and the Humors

Chapter 6 Your Humoral Calling:
  Career Choices by the Humors 105
  The Vocabulary of Humorology in Everyday Life

Chapter 7 Your Humoral Behaviors: 121
  Food, Energy, and Lifestyle by the Humors

Contents

CHAPTER 8 Your Humoral Health History: 153
    Disease Patterns by the Humors
        Modern Medicine and the Humors

CHAPTER 9 Your Humoral Balance: 165
    Making Corrections for Health, Romance, and Happiness
        The Humors in Raising Children

CHAPTER 10 Your Personal Best: 191
    Eight Archetypes of Good Humor and the Ultimate Chart
        Shakespeare and the Humors

SELECTED BIBLIOGRAPHY   213
ACKNOWLEDGMENTS   217

List of Figures

Figure 1   Basic Physiology   47
Figure 2   Physical Build   51
Figure 3   Facial Qualities   52
Figure 4   Telltale Hands   54
Figure 5   Distribution of Weight Gain   57
Figure 6   Expressing Anger   71
Figure 7   Expressing Joy   72
Figure 8   Symptoms of Imbalance   73
Figure 9   Signs of Good Balance   74
Figure 10   Key Concerns   96
Figure 11   Dominant Reaction to Conflict in a Relationship   97
Figure 12   Ways of Showing Joy in Relationships   98
Figure 13   Preferred Way of Making Up—Reconciliation   99
Figure 14   Decision-Making about Relationships   100
Figure 15   Rhythms of Relationships   101
Figure 16   Favorite Words and Phrases   102
Figure 17   Styles of Leadership   107
Figure 18   Favorite Style of Learning and
             Information Processing   109
Figure 19   Favorite Careers   118
Figure 20   Favorite Careers by the Humors—Four Men   119
Figure 21   Favorite Careers by the Humors—Four Women   120
Figure 22   Favorite Craved Foods, Flavors, and Drinks   125
Figure 23   Favorite Healthy Foods   126

List of Figures

Figure 24   The Whimsical Humors   145
Figure 25   Humorology: Summary Chart of Key Tendencies   146
Figure 26   Elemental Qualities and Environmental Influences   148

Temperamentally Yours

While reading Aristotle's *Physics,* [Thomas] Kuhn had become astonished at how "wrong" it was. How could someone who wrote so brilliantly on so many topics be so misguided when it came to physics?

Kuhn was pondering this mystery . . . when suddenly Aristotle "made sense." Kuhn realized that Aristotle invested basic concepts with different meanings than did modern physicists. Aristotle used the term *motion,* for example, to refer not just to change in position but to change in general—the reddening of the sun as well as its descent toward the horizon. Aristotle's physics, understood on its own terms, was simply different from, rather than inferior to, Newtonian physics.

Kuhn left physics for philosophy, and [wrote] *The Structure of Scientific Revolution.* The keystone of his model was the concept of a paradigm. . . . Kuhn used the term to refer to a collection of procedures or ideas that instruct scientists, implicitly, what to believe and how to work. . . . "Whenever you get two people interpreting the same data in different ways," he said, "that's metaphysics."

—JOHN HORGAN, *The End of Science* (1996), pp. 42–44

ID YOU KNOW that there is a simple way to understand yourself and your relationships that is actually more than twenty-four hundred years old and yet almost unknown today?

I sure didn't, when I was fifteen, sitting in my tenth grade English class and wondering what life was really about. Still, I had a little secret in my heart that somehow I would find a way to set an example for others to follow of how to lead a happy life of understanding and fulfillment. I was curious, eager to see how others lived and made sense of living. Travel in more than twenty countries, my parents' contribution to my education, had already shown me that the commonalities of humanity far outweighed the differences, across time as well as geography. Literature of four hundred years ago sometimes seemed as alive and real to me as anything I read in the evening paper.

So when my English teacher Mrs. Riely assigned us to do research on a particular aspect of fourteenth-century life in the time of English poet and storyteller Geoffrey Chaucer, I jumped at the chance to take a look at medieval concepts of science. I wanted to see if the ancient way of understanding life was really as quaint and useless as we, the first generation of the technological age, had been led to believe.

When I began to find out about the four temperaments and their humors and an all-encompassing philosophy of character and health that had prevailed for over two thousand years, even up to a hundred years ago, I was hooked. The ancients were on to something, I thought, something we have lost today. Some over-arching understanding of the human mind and body.

At the top of the stack of note cards I finally submitted for the project, Mrs. Riely penned in red ink, "A, Very Fine. Hold on to these—they will be useful to you for years. Occasionally you put too much on one card." I remember wondering what she could possibly be thinking. I was just having fun with some ancient metaphysics. How could it be useful to me? When I pulled out those old notes to begin this book, over thirty years later, I marveled at her prescience. Life is always more than we think.

Since then, I have filled over sixteen feet of shelf space with books about and related to the temperaments and the humors, along with eight volumes of my own notes. I believe I have dedicated more study to the humors, as my perennial hobby, than almost anyone alive except perhaps for a handful of academic experts on Paracelsus or Avicenna.

After repeated urgings by family, students, and clients over the past twenty years to write a book for them about the temperaments, I feel privileged to have had the broad experience both academically and in life necessary to be able to offer you here a taste of the richness of this ancient way of understanding character and health. Through the four temperaments and their humors and their many diverse impacts on multiple aspects of each of our lives, we can find ways of improving our health, character, romance, career, friendships, child-rearing, spiritual interests, and more. I also see now how my multidisciplined background, being a nutritionist, lawyer, family counselor, and theologian all at the same time, is not so strange as it seems, but rather places me in a unique position to fully appreciate the wisdom of the temperaments and their humors, and, I like to think, links me to a grand tradition of thinkers since ancient times who sought with the help of multiple disciplines to find a depth of understanding that allowed them to set an example of the happy life that others might follow.

I return to my question then, with which I began this introduction. Did you know that there is a simple way to understand yourself and your relationships that is more than twenty-four hundred years old and yet almost unknown today?

Did you know that even though most people have never heard of it, it was the basis of Western medical practice and character study, even into the twentieth century?

Why do some people hate to swim and others love to? Why do some people like broad-shouldered, solid physiques and others are drawn to the willowy frames? Why do some people explode with anger when others would pout and withdraw? Why do some people lead and others are content to follow? Why do some people always get colds and others never? Why does one person want an explanation for everything and another follows her gut with no questions asked?

Is it luck, genetics, environment, the stars and planets, parental conditioning, or could there be more?

When you read this book, you will discover four powerful forces that work together in important ways to determine who you are and, even more important, who you want to be. And you can find out how to use these forces and put them into balance in your life, so that you can feel, think, and act at your best, in harmony with your deepest self and also at peace with those around you. You'll know what their balance of forces is too, once you have absorbed the knowledge in this book.

These four forces have been known since before the time of Hippocrates, the most famous physician in the ancient Greek world more than two millennia ago. They were named "humors" and gave rise to four corresponding profiles among people, called "temperaments." The humors are a kind of essence, flow, force, of the universe. They were also called ethers, vapors, winds, or airs. Before chemistry and the microscope, vapors were believed to influence the body, much like energies that come and go with variations in the environment and the weather. Hippocrates associated them directly with four major liquid substances in the body.

Our present word "humor" actually comes from this ancient word. In the early European Renaissance, Europe discovered the ancient Arabian writings that had preserved the ancient Greek writings, most notably here, the Hippocratic writings, which may in turn have built upon even earlier Egyptian wisdom. The study of the influence of the four humors became something of a sensation. No less a figure than William Shakespeare both used and parodied the faddish idea of the humors and their temperaments governing a person's character and tastes—in people, places, and things. Because of the many satires in Renaissance England based on exaggerations of the prototypes of the humors and their temperaments, the term "humorous" for what had before been called "farce" and "comedy" came into vogue and is with us today, though few people know why. I've dubbed the study of the humors, "humorology."

In his book *The Traditional Healer's Handbook: A Classic Guide to the Medicine of Avicenna*, G. M. Hakim, N.D., summarizes the impact the humors this way: "The theory of humors—semivaporous substances that maintain the proper temperament of the organs— are the heart of the medicine of Hippocrates, Galen, and Avicenna, of Chinese and Ayurvedic medicine, and of virtually all other traditional systems. Yet this tremendous consensus among prominent medical authorities for two millennia is ignored."

Hearing this brief history may suggest to you how influential the humors have been down through the ages. Today most personality profiling is based on the work of Carl G. Jung, psychologist and student of psychoanalyst Sigmund Freud, who transformed the study of emotion and character into a science for the modern age. Jung was, however, also an avid student of the medieval philosopher, itinerant physician, and alchemist Paracelsus, who was a master of the art of discerning the influence of the four humors.

What does all this matter today?

The bottom line is that the profound influence of the four humors goes on today in you and me and every one of us, whether we know it or not. Not only does the science and art of the humors play a fascinating role in the art and culture of Western civilization, but also, the four humors do in fact play a huge part in our lives. As you read on and take a look at your own life, at the lives of the people you know, and at the way your relationships, preferences, career, and health unfold, you may well come to share this same conviction.

This book is intended as a handbook to help you delve into the influences of the four humors and their corresponding temperaments and begin to play with them and orchestrate them for your own greater benefit and happiness. This first book on the four temperaments and their humors in postmodern times cannot claim to be a complete working of the subject. My purpose here is to give you a tantalizing taste, to get you going, to make you aware, and to get you thinking about the humors and your own temperament, as well as those of others you know. I also invite you to use your new awareness to your advantage right away. This book will show you how.

As has been heard many times before from students in my seminars on the humors over the last twenty-five years, after you gain awareness of the humors, you will never look at other people the same way again. Or at yourself or your desires or your relationships either.

Just a reminder, this is not the idle resurrection of some unique symbolism from some lost civilization, meant to make us laugh and wonder. It is us. The most up-to-date studies of character formation, glandular function, metabolic processes, and developmental and family patterns have not contradicted in any way the conclusions drawn by keen observers of the four temperaments down through the ages. Indeed, as you will hear more about later, much contemporary science affirms the reality of these four humoral forces balancing each other, cooperating together, creating trouble and pain when out of balance, and peace and pleasure when in dynamic harmony.

Here are just a few case histories to whet your appetite for more.

Early in my career coaching with the four humors, I worked with a couple whose great results assured me I was on to something big. In our first interview, I found that the couple, Sharon and Gabe, had a number of frustrating differences. For one, they disagreed about what they should be eating. Sharon wanted a healthier diet and Gabe liked what he liked. What's more, their marriage was under stress because their sexual appetites differed drastically. He wanted sex at least every day, while a few times a month were enough for her. Once I discovered their humoral temperaments using a questionnaire like the one in Chapter 2, I was able to suggest a few dietary and lifestyle changes that could help them. They carried through, and within two weeks they called me. Gabriel's sexual appetite had mellowed and he became less strident, while Sharon's libido was reignited. They were dedicated to continuing their new dietary plan because of great results.

Another gentleman, Patrick, was a student in a continuing education course I was teaching on how to achieve your personal best using the ancient wisdom of the humors. Patrick complained that he had been trying to lose weight for over twenty years on all kinds of diets but could never be successful without constant struggle. After two weeks eating and exercising and thinking in accordance with his own humoral temperament, he reported that for the first time in decades he did not have to struggle against his appetite. He was losing weight easily and naturally and feeling better and more balanced than ever before.

A young woman I counseled named Melissa could not understand why she was repeatedly attracted to "cads," guys who were moody and emotionally distant and very difficult to deal with. Their creativity and romanticism kept blinding her to their faults. Once she had the wisdom you will find here, she could recognize these men instantly and steer away from them, or if she chose, pursue the relationship with realistic expectations, taking steps that would get the results she wanted rather than constant surprises and disappointments.

Michelle was a middle-aged woman who sought my advice with major job dissatisfaction. She made good money and got recognition for her work as a computer specialist, but something was seriously missing and it was affecting the way she treated her family. She said she was frustrated by the end of the day and had a bad attitude with her kids. We took a look at her humoral profile based on the questions I asked her, and within a month, after a few small changes you will hear about later, she felt much more satisfied and kinder to her family, even without changing her job.

My own family at one time had a very common problem. That is, cranky kids during dinner preparation time. It happened almost every night. Just when the tired parents want to relax at home and have a fun family time, the two kids are bickering at each other. With a few simple adjustments based on each person's humoral temperament, the troublesome daily scene became a time of warm family feelings and fun.

To give you an example from the business world of how powerful what you will be learning can be, I'll introduce two business partners, Sam and Mike. They complained to me in a workshop that they could never understand each other because they took such different approaches to every situation requiring a decision. Once they could appreciate each other's humoral tendencies around decision-making, they found working together much easier and more effective.

Who do you know who has struggled with difficult customers? Here is an example from the world of sales, the story of Sarah. She felt at a loss for how to appeal to the diversity of customers she approached. Only at the end of each sales pitch and after that particular customer's final objections, would she catch on to the approach she thought would have worked better for that person from the start. Once Sarah grasped the wisdom of looking for the four temperaments, she could intuit an effective approach right away. She could start off on the right foot immediately and her sales encounters were more fun and profitable. Her confidence soared.

These case histories may help you start to appreciate how enjoyable and beneficial the wisdom of the humors can be. You can reap great rewards when you can be clearer about your own needs and wants and how best to communicate them. And there is little match for the delight you can experience seeing your friends, acquaintances, and loved ones smile in recognition when you respond easily to their deepest interests and longings. With the skills you can acquire here, you can be your best self more easily and often. And you can have more influence than you thought possible at home, at work, and at leisure.

Have fun with the humors. They are not to be used to pigeon-hole yourself or anyone else. Instead let them help you spread your wings. This ancient wisdom is not meant to limit anyone's sense of his own potential, or to cause you to underestimate the reach of others. Instead it can open up new vistas and possibilities.

Whether we know it or not, we are constantly building impressions of people based on our past experience of people with similar traits. If we were bullied by a big fellow in kindergarten we may be timid around such people. But if we were befriended by a big guy, we may feel trusting and safe around them. We constantly take guesses at what other people will like. Why not make an educated guess? We all have a natural intuition about others. Why not let it be a trained intuition? If we have developed some trust in our own hunches, we are more likely to feel confident to start a conversation and actually get to know a person.

I do not know one bit of knowledge or information that cannot be misused by someone whose intentions are malevolent. This is a dilemma Albert Einstein spoke of when he told of his decision to reveal the power of the atomic nucleus. It really boils down to whether you tend to be optimistic or pessimistic about humanity. And this may depend on your temperament!

So I ask you to enjoy finding out about the temperaments in a spirit of possibility for yourself and others—an opening up. In his essay "Synergy—a Tarot Myth to Live By, Moving into the 1990s," in Greer and Pollack's *New Thoughts on Tarot* (1988), James Wanless expressed it this way: "In alchemy you take the natural ingredients—air, fire, water, and earth—and you blend them. You're the chef of your life, and your life is the soup. . . . One of the nice things about archetypal psychology like this [in alchemy and the tarot] is that not only does it bring in Jung's process of individuation, traditional psychology, as well as Eastern self-realization, mystical European alchemy, and all, but it's also fun. It's entertaining. It's fantasy—to see yourself as a Magician and watch this movie of all your different selves."

Alchemy and tarot are both derived from the ancient elements and humors, as you will see. These ancient ways of understanding are meant to increase our power and give us direction to improve our lives by all available means. Each of us was given deep passion for good in our souls, which can lead us to our greatest satisfactions and our greatest contributions. Augustine of Hippo said sixteen hundred years ago that desire is the way God steers us on our path. Probably the highest purpose to which you can apply the wisdom you will absorb here in this book is to help you and those you care about find your own individual passion and drive. This can create such a momentum of joy and discovery that your humors and your life will come into a lasting and joyful balance. You can feel that you are living every minute to your fullest—and helping others do the same. Your soul will soar as you help others soar, and you'll have the time of your life!

A note of reassurance may be helpful here. Despite the connections to alchemy and tarot and other possibly occult or mystical ways of ancient understanding, there is a long tradition of the humors in religious life. Nor do they conflict with modern scientific principles of verification.

Certainly the concept of the humors was well developed before the spiritual movements that gave rise to Christianity, Islam, and other contemporary religious beliefs. But there is a long history of acceptance of the humors by these traditions. Indeed, Hippocrates was attempting to move beyond the superstitions of his time by using the humors in his medicine. He advocated some separation of the religious world from the world of medicine, something we are very familiar with today, for better or worse, partly because of the tradition of thought Hippocrates began.

Since that time, many notable religious figures have devoted significant effort to applying the humors to increase the power of the divine in our lives. Hildegard of Bingen, a prominent nun and powerful abbess in the medieval church, wrote extensively on the humors in the twelfth century, and even went so far as to make some changes to tradition to make the male and female principles more balanced. She has become a saint in the Catholic Church. Paracelsus, writing in the early sixteenth century, was not only a physician and philosopher, but also a theologian. He developed a strong tradition still followed today among metaphysicists and students of ancient alchemy, that the true purpose of the humors and any attempt to improve the health and well-being of a person, as her physician or spiritual adviser, is to build the person's character and soul toward perfection, to take base elements and turn them to gold. Most of the scientific investigators in medicine and natural science throughout the Middle Ages were in fact supported by the church.

In more recent times, Swedenborg, Hahnemann, and Jung are just a few of the prominent figures who have comfortably combined a fascination with the ancient wisdom about the humors and health with both, on the one hand, a powerful faith in the role of the divine in health and healing and, on the other hand, a deep respect for the intellectual insights afforded by rational and scientific inquiry.

Similarly, in the Islamic world, medicine based on the humoral science of Avicenna and other Arabic physicians and scientists writing after the time of Mohammed is well respected as an integral part of the tradition of Islamic culture. For these reasons, I hope your mind is at ease that the humors can only add to and not detract from your deepest understanding as your life unfolds.

A few quick notes on how I have organized the information in this book. Chapters 1 and 2 will introduce you to the four temperaments and their underlying humors, so that you can begin to familiarize yourself with them and begin to discover your own unique balance of humors that give rise to your classic temperamental tendencies. Chapters 3 and 4 will help you explore in more detail the physical and psychological traits affected by your humors. Chapters 5 and 6 explain how your temperament and the humors affect how you relate to others in your relationships and how you relate to your work and career activities. Chapters 7 and 8 help you find out how your everyday choices and preferences are both influenced by and exert influence on the balance of your humors, with profound effects on you health and happiness. Chapters 9 and 10 show you how to make corrections for your humoral balance so that you can bring out the very best of your natural temperament for your most fulfilling and happy life.

Throughout the book you will find diagrams, charts, illustrations, and boxed textual features. Use the diagrams to obtain greater understanding of the different qualities of the humors and the corresponding temperaments. The diagrams may help you to fix in mind the contrasting characteristics represented by the humors and their various manifestations. I have adopted the spades, hearts, diamonds, and clubs symbols from playing cards in many of the diagrams as a reminder of the suggestive, unquantifiable nature of the way the humors work, as well as to remind you of how deeply the humors have penetrated our culture, how far back in history they go, and how important it is to play and have fun with them rather than let them limit or confine you.

The charts are designed to give you additional information, so that you can consider some of the ideas more deeply for yourself.

The illustrations are meant to help you grasp a mental picture of the way the humors can appear, whether in an individual or as an archetype. They are also meant to inspire your curiosity and creativity in wider application of the insights you acquire and perhaps your investigation of the many correspondences with other ways of understanding our world.

Finally, the boxed features are meant to allow for a deeper look at some concepts related to the humors without interrupting the flow of information. You can read these anytime or not at all, or refer to them to address certain questions you or others may have. Also, these features may help you to keep in mind that the study of the humors is ongoing, and everyone's living experience counts in the process. As long as you and I seek greater health, romance, and happiness, as individuals and as participants in our various families and cultures, we can hope that the physiological, psychological, social, and spiritual wisdom embodied in the humors, embedded in our personal temperaments, and rooted in the ancient cultures of the Mediterranean, can continue to fascinate us and make us ask more questions.

As scientific understanding has grown, so our world has become dehumanized. Man feels himself isolated in the cosmos, because he is no longer involved in nature and has lost his emotional "unconscious identity" with natural phenomena. These have slowly lost their symbolic implications. . . . His contact with nature has gone, and with it has gone the profound emotional energy that this symbolic connection supplied.

This enormous loss is compensated for by the symbols of our dreams. They bring up our original nature—its instincts and peculiar thinking. . . .

To be more accurate, the surface of our world seems to be cleansed of all superstitious and irrational elements. Whether, however, the real inner human world (not our wish-fulfilling fiction about it) is also freed from primitivity is another question. Is the number of 13 not still taboo for many people? . . . A realistic picture of the human mind reveals many such primitive traits and survivals, which are still laying their roles just as if nothing had happened during the last 500 years.

—CARL G. JUNG (1875–1961), "Approaching the Unconscious,"
in Jung, *Man and His Symbols,* pp. 85–86

CHAPTER 1

Your Four Humors

Now . . . in the same way that the Elements comprise the world, so too are they the fabric of the human body. And they are diffused and active throughout the body so that the body is held together, and at the same time they are spread throughout the world and work upon it. For fire, air, water, and earth are in human beings, and human beings are made from them. . . .

When the elements are properly at work in the body, they preserve it and confer health; but when they are at odds in it they weaken and kill it. For the humors, coagulated from heat, moisture, blood, and flesh in the human body, when they penetrate and remain in it and work there peacefully and in due proportion, are healthy. If, on the other hand, they reach it all at once, rushing upon it too copiously, they will weaken and destroy it. For heat and moisture and blood and flesh have all been changed, because of Adam's sin, into antagonistic humors in mankind.

—HILDEGARD OF BINGEN, *Causes and Cures,* in Flanagan,
Secrets of God: Writings of Hildegard of Bingen, (1098–1179), pp. 1151–8

T HE FOUR TEMPERAMENTS are our uniquely human way of expressing the balance of four forces that govern all things according to the ancient way of understanding character and health. These four forces are the humors, which mix and move within us and affect every aspect of our lives. They have been called influences, fluids, airs, vapors, tempers, and more. They were identified thousands of years ago, most notably in ancient Greece in the fourth century BCE, to help us interpret who we are and how we can become more of who we want to be, physically, emotionally, socially, and spiritually. The temperaments and their corresponding humors are called choleric, melancholic, sanguine, and phlegmatic, after the names used by Hippocrates, in whose medical writings the humors were fully developed as a system for health and balance. Hippocrates and his followers were famous throughout the ancient Mediterranean cultures for their pragmatism and keen observation of what kept people well and what helped them to heal. For example, he is credited with creating the diagnosis "diabetes," to describe sugar spilled in the urine, which he detected by tasting!

The humors comprise a kind of ethereal, four-corners force field that affects our physical health, our mental attitude, our romance, our career choices, and our happiness. The humors were linked to the primary elements of the universe and to the primary qualities that govern its movement. In the philosophy of Aristotle, whose conclusions about the universe dominated Western thought until the modern era, these forces were believed to reflect in the body of the person, as a divinely created microcosm, the same operational principles that are responsible for the function of the universe outside ourselves, as a divinely created macrocosm. The humors represent the powerful resonance that exists between ourselves and our surroundings, and just as our environment influences us profoundly, so do we have tremendous influence on what comes into our lives in our health, romance, and happiness.

The names of the four humors, choleric, melancholic, sanguine, and phlegmatic, sound alien and esoteric to most of us. You could invent new names for them. But then you would lose twenty-four hundred years of accumulated associations with these very names, and these associations can be helpful today. So bear with me, and see if in a little while these names can come to represent a great deal of practical information for you.

Each humor refers to a kind of fluid or flow in the body. Many researchers believe that they were never intended to directly refer to physical body substances but rather to energies that ebb and flow in harmony or competition in the body, influencing all kinds of mind and body functions.

Sanguine refers to "blood," and stands for the flow of vitality and air throughout the living system. Today we hear the term most often referring to a sanguine complexion, meaning one's face is ruddy, with blood close to the surface of the facial skin. It also sometimes refers to an optimistic outlook. The sanguine force is hot and wet in Aristotelian terms, representing the element air. Air is light and mobile, and might translate into a person whose mind, personality, or character might be described in those words. It is intriguing that as far as we know, the ancients did not know that the blood carries the air so essential to our breath and life. But nevertheless, they got the connection right.

Phlegmatic refers to the clearer fluids of the body, perhaps the fluids of the lymphatic system. We still speak of "phlegm" to refer to the thick fluids or mucus that develop when the lymphatic system and immune system are working overtime in response to a health challenge like a bacterial or fungal infection. Aristotle would characterize phlegm as cold and wet, representing the water element.

A Brief History of Humorology

THE HUMORS REFLECT a profound tradition of Western civilization: a liking for the number four as a satisfying quantity for things or categories. The four elements, humors, and temperaments at the core of ancient Greek philosophy may have its roots even earlier, among the Egyptians. In his book *The Mysteries of Osiris or Ancient Egyptian Initiation,* R. Swinborne Clymer, M.D., describes an ancient Egyptian symbology of four that goes back to the great Pyramid of Cheops. The four corners represent the four aspects of humanity—body, spirit, mind, and soul—and a balance between the male and female principles. Clymer describes the Egyptian origin for the image of the cherubim, "one of the great mysteries in the Bible," a four-faced creature represented by four beasts, described by Ezekiel as having the faces of an ox, a lion, an eagle, and a man. These four images are combined in the figure of the winged sphinx known in ancient Egypt and later Greece. These symbolic progressions and relationships were presumed in ancient times to mirror the history of the world and of the relationship between Creator and created.

Clymer believes that these beasts were originally stellar constellations visible at the commencement of the four seasons and used to predict the Nile River floods. "The ox held the winds of spring; the lion the winds of summer, " he explains. The eagle predicted the harvest, and the man foreshadowed the winter with its promise of a new beginning. Over time, this early astronomy yielded to astrology as the constellations changed and the animal images that represented them changed. Still, these symbols appear repeatedly in ancient Greek and Roman literature and again in the visions of the Prophets of the Old Testament and in references in the New Testament, and again in much cultural imagery of today. For example, in many Christian churches both ancient and modern, you can see the four Evangelists symbolized by these four creatures in many a sculpture or stained glass window, presumably intended to awaken deep archetypes of power and balance in the minds of believers.

It is still a mystery whether the Egyptians actually identified the temperaments and humors themselves, and associated these with the four directions, the four animals, or the four aspects of humanity. There is intriguing evidence that while the Greeks expanded on the Egyptian symbology in developing their concepts of the physical universe, the ancient Indian civilizations pursued the more esoteric side. It is believed, for example, that the four suits of the tarot may have come from India. These were actually outlawed in medieval Europe for being dangerously occult, suggestive of pagan arcane sciences, despite the fact that the Bible referred to many of these symbols.

It is obviously difficult to be exactly sure when the four humors were first identified, and it is tempting to postulate that all such systems can be aligned so that they correspond, especially because they so often have in common an alignment with the four ancient elements and the four directions.

In any case, we know that the temperaments, the humors, and their corresponding qualities, elements, and directions, were well known in the Golden Age of Greece, in the fourth century BCE. Hippocrates was the most famous physician of that time, made famous by his students and followers, who wrote and taught after him for almost two hundred years. He used a pragmatic approach of observation and prescription that is considered the beginning of "modern" medicine. He built his philosophy of health on the four humors as the source of imbalance and disease. A century later, Aristotle, known as the cofounder of philosophy with his teacher Plato, and as the proponent of careful observation of the physical world, built his philosophy of matter on the four elements. The Roman understanding of this ancient science was most thoroughly expounded by the famous Roman physician Galen, whose work was still revered by medical students over a thousand years later.

Much ancient wisdom was lost in the fires of Alexandria's great libraries when Egypt's capital was destroyed in Roman times. Arabic translations became the main repository for the wisdom of the ancient Mediterranean and was not accessible to European scholars until the Crusades. Meanwhile these works formed the foundation of much of the works of famous Arabic physicians Averroes and Avicenna. With the Crusades and the opening of European culture to the influences of the East, these works were brought to Europe and translated into Latin. They had several waves of influence with the ebb and flow of cultural interactions, war, or the wealth of learned benefactors. A number of medieval physicians and philosophers took up the challenge of translation, interpretation, and application. These were mostly associated with the medieval church, which patronized most scholarly work of the time.

With the European Renaissance, there was renewed secular interest in the ancient wisdom, and Renaissance healers studied the ancient texts. By the time of Elizabeth I of England, the humors were all the rage in drama as well as healing, just as language from a TV medical drama such as *ER* makes its way into everyday conversation today.

The humors held sway until the advent of modern medicine with the discovery of petrochemicals and the pharmaceuticals that could be made from them in the laboratory.

Water hugs the ground but is powerfully irresistible, and might be metaphorical for a person of such a character.

Choleric refers to the bile, the yellowish fluid produced in the digestive system to help absorb digested nutrients. We are most familiar today with the root of this word in the current term "cholesterol," referring to a fatty substance found in the bile. Cholesterol is necessary for a number of body functions, such as digestion, immune factors, and hormone production. It is feared today because it is found to accumulate in damaged arterial vessels. The choleric humor gone awry can be responsible for such problems, as you will hear in Chapter 8. According to Aristotle's theories of matter, the choleric force is hot and dry, representing the element of fire. Fire is warm and all-encompassing. It can stand for a person whose charisma and energy is undeniable.

Melancholic refers to the "black bile," and to this day, in the contemporary mode of examining the body, we're not quite sure what physical fluid this might actually correspond to. My hunch is that we just don't want to talk about it in our post-Victorian squeamishness. It probably refers to the stool, the dark material that moves from the thirty feet of small intestine into the large intestine to be expertly sorted out there, the useful materials from the waste, so that the latter can be expelled pronto from the body. The melancholic force is cool and dry in Aristotelian terms, representing the element of the earth in our bodies. It might be thought of as that transformation of food into life plus waste, the latter then made available for other organisms to transform into more life. The element of earth is supremely creative of life and responsive to air and water but has a cool demeanor. I am sure you can imagine someone like that.

Hardly a system to build two thousand years of wisdom on! you might think. But please don't judge too soon. It has been done, so let's see what validity it may hold for us today.

Air, water, fire, and earth are a foursome you may have come across before if you have looked into astrology or other esoteric sciences of the ancient Mediterranean world. This connection can instantly enrich what you read here about the humors.

According to this ancient art and science, the four humors are present in your body and mine and everyone else's. They become most interesting when you come to realize ten basic facts about the humors.

[1] *Unique balance.* You and every other person tend to have your own unique balance of the four humors.

[2] *One dominates.* One humor has a slight dominance at the core of every person, physically, mentally, emotionally, and spiritually, and gives rise to one of four archetypal temperaments.

[3] *Discomfort from imbalance.* Whenever outside conditions, your own decisions or actions, or your internal responses to conditions cause a departure from your own natural balance, you will experience discomfort either directly or indirectly.

[4] *Deliberate rebalancing.* By altering outside conditions, your decisions or actions, or your internal responses to conditions, you can return yourself to balance and to a more happy, comfortable state.

[5] *Natural tendency to balance.* Your body naturally tends to bring itself back into humoral balance, and many surprising and sometimes undesirable choices are attempts to achieve this rebalancing.

[6] *Chronic conditions call for support of all humors.* If a problem is chronic and persistent, chances are good that your dominant humor is overstimulated and exhausted or depleted, because too much has been demanded of it. It will need deep regeneration for you to achieve true health, along with nourishment of the other humors.

[7] *Acute conditions call for focus on the dominant humor.* If a problem is sudden and acute, chances are good that your dominant humor may need a temporary nudge of a healthy kind to put you back on track.

[8] *Excessive humor.* From time to time you may be exposed to too much of another humor, and this will require careful rebalancing.

[9] *Empowerment.* Conscious awareness of how the humors operate empowers you to avoid health-damaging, temporary fixes or craved substitutes and to embrace health-giving, deeply enjoyable solutions to any problem in your life.

[10] *Helping others.* Not only can you rebalance yourself with this knowledge for greater health and happiness, but you can also help others feel more comfortable, healthy, and creative by staying aware of their humoral needs.

That's it in a nutshell—the art of the four temperaments and their humors. So lets get on with it! What's your humor?

※

For the sun and the moon and all planets, as well as all the stars and the whole chaos, are in man. . . . The body attracts heaven . . . and this takes place in accordance with the great divine order. Man consists of the four elements, not only—as some hold—because he has four tempers, but also because he partakes of the nature, essence, and properties of the elements. . . .

Consider how great and noble man was created, and what greatness must be attributed to his structure! No brain can fully encompass the structure of man's body and the extent of his virtues; he can be understood only as an image of the macrocosm, of the Great Creature. Only then does it become manifest what is in him. For what is outside is also inside; and what is not outside man is not inside. The outer and the inner are *one* thing, *one* constellation, *one* influence, *one* concordance, *one* duration . . . *one* fruit.

—PARACELSUS (1493–1541), "The Book Paragranum,
Revised in Four Books," in Jacobi, *Paracelsus: Selected Writings*, p. 21

CHAPTER 2

What's Your Humor?

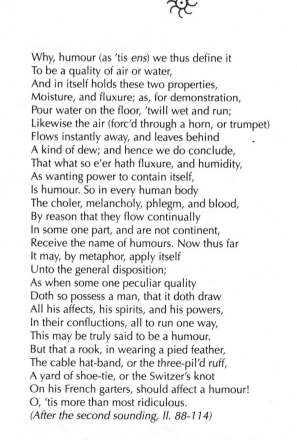

Why, humour (as 'tis *ens*) we thus define it
To be a quality of air or water,
And in itself holds these two properties,
Moisture, and fluxure; as, for demonstration,
Pour water on the floor, 'twill wet and run;
Likewise the air (forc'd through a horn, or trumpet)
Flows instantly away, and leaves behind
A kind of dew; and hence we do conclude,
That what so e'er hath fluxure, and humidity,
As wanting power to contain itself,
Is humour. So in every human body
The choler, melancholy, phlegm, and blood,
By reason that they flow continually
In some one part, and are not continent,
Receive the name of humours. Now thus far
It may, by metaphor, apply itself
Unto the general disposition;
As when some one peculiar quality
Doth so possess a man, that it doth draw
All his affects, his spirits, and his powers,
In their confluctions, all to run one way,
This may be truly said to be a humour.
But that a rook, in wearing a pied feather,
The cable hat-band, or the three-pil'd ruff,
A yard of shoe-tie, or the Switzer's knot
On his French garters, should affect a humour!
O, 'tis more than most ridiculous.
(After the second sounding, ll. 88-114)

—ASPER, speaking in Ben Jonson, *Everyman Out of His Humour* (1599),
in Dutton, *Ben Jonson: To the First Folio*, p. 35

WHAT IS YOUR humor? What cluster of qualities help make you the unique person you are? You will get a quick handle on which is most likely your dominant humor when you have completed this eighteen-point questionnaire. Notice what a variety of characteristics are involved. The humors touch every aspect of life.

And notice the variety of responses possible to each question. Awareness of the humors often helps us appreciate the diversity among people, even those close to us. Even though we all want basically the same things, to be comfortable and free of pain, to love and be loved, to feel alive and unafraid, we each go about achieving these things in our own unique ways.

Feel free to answer this questionnaire on your own or with a friend or family member or group. It can be a good deal of fun to hear how others may characterize you or how they characterize themselves.

Your
Temperament
Questionnaire

[1] My basic skeletal structure might best be characterized as
- **C** squarish, solid, robust, larger than average for my sex
- **P** rounded, childlike, smaller than average
- **m** willowy, long, delicate, tall
- **S** angular, curvy, compact
- **U** can't decide (ask a friend)

[2] My facial features include mostly
- **m** oval shape, shallow set, open eyes, even front teeth, wide smile, high cheekbones, high forehead
- **S** heart shape, deep-set eyes, small mouth, crowded teeth, small pointed chin, forehead narrowing towards top, widow's peak at hairline
- **C** Squarish shape, broadish forehead, big teeth, squared jaw, rounded eyes relatively close together
- **P** rounded face, small teeth, youthful smile, rounded cheeks, almond eyes
- **U** can't decide (ask a friend!)

[3] When (and if) I put on weight, it goes mostly to my
- **S** outside of thighs, inside of thighs, pear shape
- **m** back of upper arms and butt, hourglass shape, belly in men
- **C** waist, back of shoulders, breasts in women, neck in men, inverted pear
- **P** all over, knees, face, apple shape
- **U** can't decide (don't ask a friend! You don't want to know what they have noticed!)

[4]   My hands are mostly
  s   small, short, would never make it in a nail polish ad
  m   one of my best features, long, tapered
  c   big, squarish, good for handshake
  P   delicate, small
  U   can't decide (compare with some friends)

[5]   When I get angry, I tend to
  c   take over, win through intimidation
  s   argue, persuade, convince, jabber on, bluster, bombast
  m   deny, accuse, blame, withdraw, sulk
  P   pout, act out, yell, cry, complain
  U   can't decide (ask a close friend)

[6]   When I am happy and excited I tend to
  P   exclaim, want to play and laugh with good friends
  m   want to celebrate, get creative, dance, sing, often by
       myself
  c   feel superconfident, plan big things, enroll others in my
       vision
  s   want to throw a party, get others to feel the same way
  U   don't know, maybe never feel that way (with awareness of
       your humors you soon will!)

[7]   If someone I just met is nasty to me, I am most likely to
  s   respond with sarcasm and hope not to meet them again
  m   go out of my way to avoid them
  c   tell them off mightily
  P   give them a second chance
  U   can't decide

[8]   My favorite snack foods fall mostly into this category
  c   salted peanuts, chips, or a quick hamburger
  m   sweets, chocolate, bread, sugar, cookies
  s   buttery pastries, cheesecake, cinnamon buns, gingerbread
       and cream cheese
  P   milk, cheese, fruit, sweetened yogurts
  U   never snack (good, but if you did . . .)

[9] The kind of exercise I like most is

   C   highly competitive

   m   fast moving, with lots of variety

   S   self-regulated, on my own, rhythmic

   P   with a group, noncompetitive

   U   never exercise (you will when you know more about what you want as a result of knowing your humors)

[10] I am attracted to men who appear

   P   big and strong with wide forehead, big chest, powerful look

   S   tall and wiry with tall forehead, intellectual look

   C   smaller and youthful looking with rounded features, smiling eyes

   m   shorter and athletic-looking with well-formed butt, may have early hairline recession, intellectual look

   U   love them all (try to discern a preference!)

[11] I am attracted to women who appear

   S   shapely, tall, and big-breasted with narrow ankles, long fingers

   m   medium build and hour-glass figured with delicate facial features

   P   strong and athletic-looking with wide shoulders, small hips

   C   small and youthful-looking with rounded face and body

   U   love them all (try to discern a preference!)

[12] My ideal career would be more like

   C   leading a top-notch corporation or organization

   S   teaching people how to enjoy all that life has to offer

   m   creating a masterpiece of art, literature, or culture

   P   helping people overcome challenges in different areas of their lives

   U   don't have a clue (what do you like most about your current work?)

[13] Success for me is closest to

    P   having a rewarding family life

    C   being all I can be, a leader's leader

    S   setting an example to others of extraordinary living

    m   getting the most out of life

    U   don't know (you will soon)

[14] The pattern of my ideal day is closest to

    m   sleep late, lively after breakfast, sleepy after lunch, sometimes stay up late

    S   sleep consistently, love mornings and evenings

    C   sleep less than most people, going all day, relax early evening

    P   lots of sleep, early to bed, enjoy daytime best

    U   can't decide (ask spouse or relative)

[15] My tendency with meals is

    C   I like a big protein breakfast and dinner, not big on sweets

    S   I love breakfast, could skip dinner, like small protein meals

    P   I don't pay much attention to meals, eat fruit, pasta, and dairy, not eggs

    m   I eat a light breakfast if any, like a large lunch, eat muffins, pasta, bagels, or vegetables for snacks

    U   can't tell

[16] My favorite weather and time of year is:

    S   warm and wet, spring, flowers and trees blooming all over, time of sowing, rebirth

    m   cold and dry, autumn, time of harvest, between the summer heat and the solitude of winter

    C   hot and dry, summer, everything in glorious fullness, most active, alive time

    P   cold and wet, winter, quiet, cold breezes, cozy family feeling

    U   no opinion (knowing your humor will help you come to embrace lots of things more consciously that really make you feel good!)

[17] I pay best attention when things come to me by way of:

P   touch—"Show me, can I touch it, hold it?" "That really touches me!"

m   sound—"Let me hear your opinion and then I'll tell you." "I hear you, that sounds right to me."

s   smell/taste—"Let me just see how it feels." "It feels right to me!"

c   sight—"I'll believe it when I see it." "Let's just see." "I can see it now! I see, I see."

v   don't know (If someone shows you a flower by the road, what do you do?)

[18]   When I make a decision:

m   I think long and hard to decide what is the best course and often reexamine my choice if there are any glitches but defend my choice actively against others' opinions.

P   I take my time, gather opinions, and then make my choice, and may reconsider if trusted friends advise caution

s   I make a quick assessment, wait for a sense of intuition, decide, and then stick with it, but remain flexible about little things

c   I make quick decisions, go with my gut, and rarely look back

v   undecided (maybe P?)

Thank you for completing all eighteen questions. If you have not done these yet, do go back and complete them now. Without this baseline of your own responses based on humoral traits, reading on will have far less value and meaning for you. Even if you are most interested in how a family member or friend would respond to these questions, knowing what your own responses are will give you much better insight into the humors of the other person.

The Ancient
Masters of the Humors

CERTAIN HISTORICAL FIGURES stand out in the history of the humors. We can trace a direct line of transmission across some twenty-four hundred years through their biographies. The real giants are six: Hippocrates, Aristotle, Galen, Avicenna, Hildegard of Bingen, and Paracelsus, because they left the most extensive expositions of the art, and because they can inspire us today with their creativity and willingness to build on what went before. For example, Hildegard of Bingen went against tradition in describing the hierarchy of elements, because she did not believe that both of the masculine-tempered elements should be higher than both of the feminine-tempered elements.

EMPEDOCLES, C. 450 BCE

Greek scientist who is credited with proposing four substances as the fabric of the universe.

HIPPOCRATES, C. 460–377 BCE

Greek physician, "father of modern medicine." He practiced on the Greek island of Cos and was a famous teacher of physicians. He and his followers composed a collection of seventy-two writings over two centuries. He was known for his careful observation, diagnosis, and prognosis, which contrasted to more magical forms of healing practiced until then. He believed that the four humors were responsible for disease in the body. He expounded on their influences, on ways to diagnose their imbalances, and on ways to promote healing through control of the humors.

ARISTOTLE, 384–322 BCE

Greek philosopher and scientist, son of the court physician to King Philip of Macedonia, who was to be grandfather of world conqueror Alexander the Great, who in turn became a student of Aristotle. Aristotle had been a student of Plato, who was a student of Socrates. He taught in Plato's Academy. He wrote on physics, logic, metaphysics, biology, rhetoric, politics, psychology, and more, including *Categories: Letters to Alexander on the World System.* Much of what we have is from notes from his lectures. His descriptions of the four elements of fire, air, water, and earth, which in particular combinations compose all things, have been fundamental to much of metaphysical thought in the medieval, Arabic, and later Western tradition.

GALEN (CLAUDIUS GALENUS), c. 130–201 CE

Greek physician, born in Asia Minor, physician to gladiators, later friends and physician to the Roman emperor and philosopher Marcus Aurelius, and then two subsequent emperors. He wrote voluminously, including fifteen commentaries on Hippocrates. He was the first to diagnose using the pulse. His work was the standard medical text for many centuries, until the advent of modern science. His writings on the humors were largely responsible for their use in ancient Rome and their rediscovery in Renaissance times by way of Arabic translations reintroduced to Europe after the Crusades.

BOETHIUS, c. 480–524 CE

Roman philosopher, commentator on Aristotle, Roman consul, and a chief minister, later executed for treason. During his imprisonment he wrote one of the most widely read books of all time, on the consolation of philosophy. His work served to validate and perpetuate the central place of Aristotle in natural philosophy.

AVICENNA (HAKIM IBN SINA), 980–1037 CE

Arabic physician and philosopher, and main interpreter of Aristotle to the Islamic world. Famous for his learning and many writings, he was physician to several sultans and a vizier in Persia. His textbook *Canon of Medicine* was a standard text for centuries. His work was a principal vehicle for the reintroduction of the ancient Greek traditions of Hippocratic medicine, and specifically the humors, to western Europe.

Averroes (ibn Rushd), 1126–98 ce

Most famous of Islamic philosophers, writer on jurisprudence and medicine, as well as philosophy. Court physician to Caliph Abu Yusuf. His most influential work was *Commentaries on Aristotle*. His was another major vehicle of transmission between the Greek doctors and the science of Renaissance Europe.

Hildegard of Bingen, 1098–1179 ce

Visionary, physician, head of a convent in medieval Germany whose advice was sought by major heads of state throughout Europe on politics and health. She might also be described as the first gynecologist. She wrote many treatises, on her visions, on women's and marital health, and on the humoral system of medicine, as well as on theological and cosmological topics. Most notable regarding the humors was her *Causes and Cures,* describing her overall cosmology based on the four elements as well as some two hundred disease conditions and recommended treatments.

Albertus Magnus, 1193–1280 ce

German philosopher, mentor to Thomas Aquinas. Student of zoology, botany, and the Aristotelian, Arabic, Jewish, and Neoplatonic traditions of astronomy, geography, and medicine. Author of many treatises, including *Of Effects in Nature*. Again affirms the validity of the traditional humoral view of human health.

Geoffrey Chaucer, c. 1345–1400 ce

First great English poet, became the standard for written English. Served in the king's household, traveled much of Europe, most famous work is the *Canterbury Tales,* c. 1386. His lively portraits of characters from his time give a unique impression of late medieval Europe and the knowledge, beliefs, and science, including that of the humors, prevalent at that time.

PARACELSUS, OR PHILIPPUS AUREOLUS THEOPHRASTUS BOMBAST VON HOHENHEIM, 1493–1541 CE

Swiss/German alchemist and physician, itinerant teacher. Studied minerals and mining diseases in particular, and various chemical compounds. Wrote in detail about humoral medicine and sought to improve upon it. The name he gave himself means "beyond Celsus," famous first-century Roman physician whose medical writings were among the first to be printed in 1478 and whose name we know from his work with the thermometer. Paracelsus' exposition of the humors is exhaustive, but he too added to what went before. He criticized blind reliance on the humoral adjustments to the exclusion of more intuitive, spiritual, and religious elements of healing. He is considered the quintessential alchemist of medieval Europe, his goal being not to transmute base metal into gold but to transmute base character into an enlightened one, that is, to heal the soul.

After you have completed the questions, you may have noticed what a wide variety of characteristics were included, and also what a range of responses are possible. The humoral tendencies represent clusters of traits. You will see as you read more that every willowy creature isn't a born artist or every large squarish figure a born leader. But according to the humors, there's a very good probability that he is exactly that, or will turn out to be as his true calling emerges and greater happiness enters into his life.

Let's go on to scoring, so you will have an idea of your dominant humor, your temperament, and the balance to which you constitutionally tend. Then we'll see why each question means what it does.

Simply count up the number of answers you marked C (choleric), S (sanguine), P (phlegmatic), or M (melancholic). The one for which you marked the most answers is your dominant humor, by your natural inclination. The second highest number is your subdominant humor, which can take over if your dominant one is depleted or overstressed to exhaustion. The lowest score is your weakest humor. Surprising breakthroughs can happen when you give a little extra attention to that humor. For example, people who befuddle you may all of a sudden make a bit more sense. And the next lowest score may be kind of an anchor humor that you take for granted, but still it could use occasional focused attention for optimal balance in your life.

Chances are that your least dominant humor is P if you are C, and C if you are P. Likewise, if you are M or S, your least dominant humor is probably S or M. You will be finding out in a later chapter why this is so.

In most cases, after you have your totals, you will find that you have at least eight or nine answers in one category. No matter how balanced anyone is, there is one humor that dominates as a physiological fact, as you will hear more about later. If you seem to be perfectly balanced, two things may be at work. On the positive side, you may be in very healthy balance, able to appreciate and maximize the gifts of your dominant humor while keeping the others well empowered in order to respond flexibly to various different situations. On the negative side, you may be trying too hard to be balanced, perhaps to the point of denying some intrinsic gifts and preferences that if allowed to be maximized would bring you greater satisfaction, happiness, and effectiveness in your life.

If it appears that two humors are vying for dominance of your temperament, the subordinate humor may be a close second and take over at times, such as when the dominant gland is exhausted. But in my experience and the interpretations of many others, there is just one that is the preferred source of vitality under stress. It is most obvious in our childhood preferences, before we have learned what we "should" like, and in our physiology, where the humors manifest most visibly because of their influences during our development.

When it appears that two are equal, it pays to explore further and check other characteristics of the person. Sometimes the most telling items are the most intimate, like your frequency of sexual desire in young adulthood, or your most secret dreams of your perfect career. For example, would you most like to be a triumphant general, a great novelist, a famous orator, or a frontier doctor? Another telling question is, what is your grandest fantasy of contribution to the future of the world? For example, would you most like to imagine yourself as the power behind a president, the composer of music that moves nations to freedom, the negotiator of a workable system to end all war, or the discoverer of a cure for a major debilitating disease? Use these more subtle and less quantifiable but more intuitive discernments to break a tie. By the way, both questions are in the C, M, S, and P order.

You may wonder whether your innate humor tendencies can change or shift over time. Essentially, no. You have one temperament that is yours, at least since birth. The humors can be manipulated and distorted severely though, most often by poor diet, inadequate rest, work that doesn't suit you, or addictions. As soon as these are corrected, your true nature will reemerge.

It is beautiful to watch the peace that comes when a person finally discovers her true temperament. There is always an aha! A sigh of acceptance and joy. If you don't feel that way about the way you come out on the questionnaire or the charts in this book, keep up the exploration until you do feel that way. It's only a matter of time and effort. Keep tweaking the various variables until you discover who you really are and want to be.

Another frequently asked question is whether humoral tendencies are inherited. There is definitely an inheritable tendency toward a particular humor or pattern of humors. Children almost always take after one or the other parent. Adopted children may adopt the behaviors and preferences of one or both parents, but until they find their own, they may feel a bit disoriented. Severe dietary distortion or other stress in pregnancy or infancy may change a person's humor by creating permanent damage to the physiological functions that modulate a particular humor, but this is rare.

It is likely that different ethnic groups around the world once tended toward different dominant humors, and this has been studied in the past by such researchers as Weston A. Price and Melvin Page, whose works are indeed fascinating (see the Bibliography). But in North America and other developed countries, for all practical purposes, ethnic background cannot be relied on. The ethnic gene pools here have long since given up their homogeneity, having mixed for several and often many generations. In the latest census of 2000, a large minority of responders chose to answer "none of the above" or "multiracial" to questions about their ethnic group. You can't therefore count on any assumptions about any individual's humoral tendencies based on historical ethnic lines.

This may give rise to another issue. What accounts for such diverse and distinct dietary preferences across ethnic cultures? How can the humors work for everyone in that culture? Are some condemned to be out of balance?

It is fascinating to study exactly what each culture develops as its favorite cuisine to suit its geographical homeland and the flora and fauna available there. It's an urgent science to document all these patterns, because few cultures today even remember, much less practice, all the complementary components of their cuisine. Nor do they live in their original habitat, where the plants and animals offered a complementary mix from which to develop the cuisine in the first place. Anthropologists have argued about meat or no meat, milk or no milk, how much of each major mineral, how much fiber, how much protein or carbohydrate, and so on. But too often they have ignored the favored condiments, herbs, and spices of each culture and the special processes different foods are subjected to by way of tradition. Yet these processes often either deactivate poisons or bring out certain valuable nutritional factors while maintaining the nutritional and enzyme integrity of the foods.

To use one example, when native Americans were first studied, the experts marveled at how well they did on a diet that was so heavy on corn, when corn was so low in minerals. Much later they discovered that the tribe being studied routinely mixed ash from a cactus plant with the corn mash and significantly increased the mineral content of the corn dish. When asked what they ate, of course they said corn, but for them corn meant corn properly prepared, with the ash their ancestors had always used. Why would they bother to mention it? Today anthropologists try to spend days and weeks right with the cooks to see exactly what goes on, but in some cultures this just is not acceptable for traditional social reasons.

It is known that in traditional cultures where the populations are still healthy, with good developmental bone structure, fertility until late ages, pleasant demeanor, and robust health into advanced age, to name a few key variables, meals are steeped in tradition, very important and very sociable, with lots of variety and freedom to eat exactly what you want and how much you want.

In addition, possibly most important of all, even though many traditional foods are carefully processed for safety and digestibility, there are rarely any foods in these diets that are highly concentrated by the removal of their water and fiber. This is in stark contrast to the typical fast-food diet in developed nations, where often over half of our calories come from foods whose natural water and fiber have been removed, and with them the majority of natural vitamins and minerals. Yet these missing factors can be just the ticket for putting the body in the best position for balancing the humors. Each mineral and vitamin can have an impact, which will have to wait for another book, and natural vegetable and fruit juices in the plant itself help balance the humors nicely, because they give the person exactly what the body expected to get when it felt a desire for that food.

For example, if a child from a traditional tribe wants something sweet, she will search for a fruit. With that sweet flavor, she will get water, fiber, minerals, and vitamins, all of which nourish her humors by way of the glands that affect her energy and growth patterns. A modern child who reaches for a candy gets purified sugar that unnaturally boosts the thyroid gland and sets her up for melancholia later. She also gets artificial colorings and flavorings that will stress the liver and add to her melancholia. Which sounds more civilized, really?

Now that you have an idea of your basic balance of humors, we'll go into each of these dimensions of the humors in detail and show you how you can find quick solutions to problems both big and small. If as occasionally can happen, you decide you have not gotten a true answer from the above questionnaire, don't despair. As you learn more about the humors, you may find that you are learning more about yourself, and you might answer one or more of the questions differently next time around.

Western biochemical medicine endeavors to trace each of these complex chemical interactions, ultimately to discover when and where one or more of the biochemical exchanges are amiss. . . . Traditional healing, while taking some interest in these complex biochemical interactions, holds that ultimately we cannot know the total interworkings of the human body. There are many religious references to the fact that the human body has been created "infinitely more complex than the entire universe." (Hadith). Therefore, the Tibb system [Arabic holistic medicine, codified by Avicenna] retreats to a comprehensible stance, which evaluates food and diet in terms of their ability to enhance or impede *metabolism*. . . .

A great many factors and considerations follow from the above, but one of the most important is that foods should be selected that (a) are in accord with the temperament of the individual and appropriate to the season, age, climate, etc.; and (b) produce balance in the four humors.

The key concept-word in Tibb is *temperament (mizaj)*. . . . While admitting the existence of microbes, the Tibb system claims that it is the *original imbalance of temperament* that provides an altered biotic environment in which these viruses and bacteria can thrive.

—HAKIM G. M. CHISHTI, N.D. *The Traditional Healer's Handbook:*
A Classic Guide to the Medicine of Avicenna, p. 19

CHAPTER 3

Your Humoral Physique:
Physical Traits by the Humors

Man emerged from the first matrix, the maternal Womb of the Great World. . . . [H]e received his material body from earth and water. These two elements constitute the body in its transient, animal life, which man as a natural being received from divine creation. . . . For we must know that man has two kinds of life—animal life and sidereal [governed by the fixed stars, of heaven] life. . . . Hence man has also an animal body and a sidereal body, and both are one, and are not separated. The relations between the two are as follows. The animal body, the body of flesh and blood, is in itself always dead. Only through the action of the sidereal body does the motion of life come into the other body. The sidereal body is fire and air; but it is also bound to the animal life of man. Thus mortal man consists of water, earth, fire, and air.

—PARACELSUS (1493-1541), "The Three Books of the *Opus Paramirum*,"
Jacobi, *Paracelsus: Selected Writings*, p. 18

OW THAT YOU have a good idea of your innate temperament and your humoral balance, let's look at what you can do with this information—what your natural humoral tendencies are in more detail—based on the ten facts listed in Chapter I. Not only can the humors help you to understand yourself, others, and your relationships better, but they can also help you identify problems quickly and find doable and lasting solutions, often where others would least expect to find them. The trick is to get the humors back in balance. They are always shifting and changing, so you will do well to think of it as a dynamic balance. That's normal—part of life. But if things feel wrong, check for balance in the humors and you'll know just what to do. It may be as simple as a hot shower or a cold swim!

It seems a stretch to believe that some antiquated concept of bodily influences could actually have an impact on our personal build and physique. Aren't we too advanced scientifically to waste our time on such an imprecise approach?

The facts are such that these humors can still today explain as much about our physical development as any other system of analysis except for simply looking at your parents and grandparents and concluding, "Yes, you do take after your mother."

A number of physical traits tend to cluster together in different people. You probably know this unconsciously, intuitively, just from observing people since childhood, but like most people, you have given it little conscious thought. For example, rarely will a tall gentleman with large shoulders and forehead have a petite mouth and full lips. Nor will a lanky ballerina-type lady have large squarish hands. Only with computer simulations and possibly plastic surgery can these things happen. But when we see it, something tells us it is odd, unnatural.

Even if there are clusters of characteristics that we all intuitively recognize and expect, you may wonder, is it not arbitrary to connect them to the four humors of ancient natural philosophy?

There are two answers here. One is this: the art of the humors was useful for two thousand years and has proven a help to physicians, psychologists, and even career counselors to the present day. So perhaps we can suspend disbelief for a time simply out of respect for prior human experience until we see what insights we might get from this inquiry.

The second answer is this: Recent scientific investigation does suggest concrete chemical and biological mechanisms that can explain the link between the humors and physical developmental traits.

In the first half of the twentieth century, Melvin Page did extensive study of the influence of endocrine function, that is hormone production, by certain important glands in the body. He found different glandular hormones tended to dominate in different populations, resulting in different physical traits. For example, he found that populations tending to have high pituitary hormone levels in their bodies during the developmental years relative to other hormones, from a high consumption of dairy for generations, tended toward a certain classic physique that was on the short side, with rounded features and fat accumulation fairly equally over the whole body but noticeably around the knees. This happens to correspond closely to the characteristics of the phlegmatic dominant humoral type.

There now seems to be good reason to believe the identification of the four humors in ancient times may correspond roughly to the four glandular or hormonal systems that most affect the development of your physique, especially from ages seven to fourteen. These four hormonal influences have their effects especially as mediated through our energy production systems under stress.

For example, if you are feeling stressed, your body tends to rely on extra hormone stimulation to get you through the stress. You may well be familiar with the adrenal glands as the "stress glands." Their fight or flight response is well known. But stress can call on other hormones. While I might rely on my sex hormones to give me a boost, someone else might look to a push from the thyroid hormones. The habitual preference of each person over the years of development largely determines their physiology. And the ancient observers who could not even detect a hormone because they didn't have the microscope or the chemistry, were still able to see that there were four dominant patterns to human development.

Notice in Figure I how the four humors correspond to the four endocrine glands that produce the hormones that control our body functions in close cooperation with our nervous system. You will hear more detail about the glandular connection when we talk about diet and health.

I have found this four-quarter diagram to be most helpful in offering a simple way to help visualize the various dimensions and influences of the humors, so you can compare and contrast them. Each diagram will add to your understanding and familiarity with the humors, so that you will develop a trained intuition about the humors and the temperaments to which they give rise.

For these diagrams, I have included the suit symbols from the common playing card deck, to stimulate your imagination about possible correspondences and to resonate with the cultural symbols your mind might play with. In her book *Tarot Mirrors: Reflections of Personal Meaning,* Mary Greer writes, "Not all taroists agree as to which element corresponds to which suit. The important thing is to trust the system you use. Through time, experience, and observation your system will work for you whatever its correspondences."

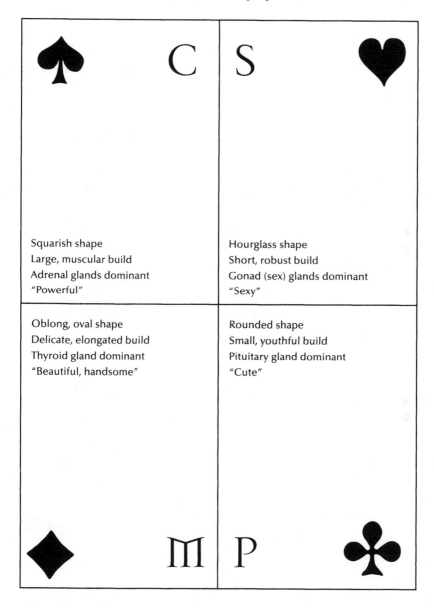

Squarish shape
Large, muscular build
Adrenal glands dominant
"Powerful"

Hourglass shape
Short, robust build
Gonad (sex) glands dominant
"Sexy"

Oblong, oval shape
Delicate, elongated build
Thyroid gland dominant
"Beautiful, handsome"

Rounded shape
Small, youthful build
Pituitary gland dominant
"Cute"

FIGURE 1. **Basic Physiology.** The dominant impression you would get in first seeing a person of each temperament is described here, along with the glandular system which tends to dominate that person's physiological development and energy metabolism when under stress. When trying to determine someone's temperament, it's best to use overall impressions first and last, using more specific traits during your assessment, when you're not sure.

The Humors and the Playing Cards

THE FOUR HUMORS are directly related to the suits of the playing cards and, in turn, to the four suits of the tarot. The history of tarot is very murky but experts maintain there are hints of it going back to ancient Egypt. Hard science can only trace it back a few hundred years to medieval Europe and possibly ancient India. Part of the reason for the mystery is that the medieval Roman church in Europe forbade the tarot and all playing with the cards because they were considered pagan witchcraft, a form of divination or fortune-telling that the church frowned upon. The use of the cards went underground but persisted all over Europe, many say through the independent gypsy tribes who roamed Europe. These were some of the few nomads remaining after medieval Europe was fenced in.

Our present playing cards are an evolutionary step from the tarot. They are all that's left after the original allegorical cards, usually twenty-two, were eliminated. The medieval Church was successful in preventing the use of all but the fifty-two cards, leaving out the more interesting "face" cards of the tarot.

It seems that whenever you retrieve ancient wisdom and apply it to modern life, there is controversy about how things match up, since each person's experience is different. This subject is no exception. There is some controversy about how the tarot suits match up with the ancient elements, and there is even some controversy about how the suits of the modern playing cards match up with the tarot suits, since these two traditions evolved separately for several hundred years before experts tried more recently to bring them back together.

The generally accepted position among mainstream tarot experts links the tarot suits with the elements as follows: the wand with sun (choleric), sword with air (sanguine), pentacle with earth (melancholic), and chalice with water (phlegmatic). Though the issue is still not settled, many experts believe that for the everyday playing cards, the spades link to the wand, the hearts to the air, the diamonds to the earth, and the clubs to the water.

There is so much symbolism throughout the history of the last twenty-four hundred years as well as multiple associations in our own common-sense impressions, that almost any point of view can be argued.

For example, why sword with air? A sword cuts air, but it also means power, a choleric trait. And a chalice holds water, but it also can hold the blood of life that carries the breath of life—the air—throughout the body. Perhaps the club is a powerful weapon of the dominant personality of the choleric instead of a symbol of water. Everyone seems clear that the diamond goes with the pentacle and the earth, but many are not sure what the pentacle symbol is in the first place.

Perhaps, when the tarot became so controversial and the medieval church wanted to outlaw fortune-telling and fortune-tellers, the playing cards persisted on by deliberately confusing and hiding the direct links of the suits we use today in our card decks with the traditional tarot suits. Yet today, many people "tell their fortunes" using everyday playing card decks. As any tarot expert or fortune-teller will tell you, much of what they do is to fine-tune their gift of intuition through use of the cards, so that the exact accuracy of their understanding of the symbols is not as important as their openness to the insights and wisdom that can come to them in focused attention to deeper wisdom. (See also the Ultimate Chart in the last chapter).

I have based my interpretations on sound opinion in the field, along with my own experience in interpreting people's health with the use of the elements and the humors. I have used the playing card suit symbols in the diagram squares to emphasize that the humoral symbols are subconsciously all around us, and that we may be using them whether we know it or not.

For example, just to take one thought, what does it mean to have a hierarchy of suits in our everyday games? Spades, hearts, diamonds, clubs? Does the order have subtle or not so subtle implications? What suit do you most identify with, or which did you like best as a kid, on a purely gut level? Does that have anything to do with your dominant humor, your temperament, and who you are, really?

I suggest that it does. Every one of us is fully ourselves in every little decision or passing preference we express. It's fun, at the very least, to explore these things. And it can be a source of powerful insight, as it has been for thousands of people whom I have watched play with the humors and their symbols.

You can have a lot of fun trying to capture the essence of a person's physique as it manifests his own particular temperament and balance of humors. For example, if you were to meet a person in any of these groups who was a perfect prototype for their dominant gland (and you will, if you look), the one-word descriptions in Figure I might easily come to mind.

Figure I summarizes the key physical characteristics of the four temperaments. The sanguine is smaller than average build, solid of shape, rounded behind, small but angular shoulders, shorter than average neck, with shapely legs and arms.

The choleric and melancholic are usually on the taller side, the choleric being more squarish of build, with broad shoulders and relatively straight hips and legs and torso.

The melancholic has a more delicate, smaller boned frame, with more sloped shoulders, small wrists and ankles, long leg bones and lengthy neck.

The phlegmatic is often the shortest of the temperamental types, with rounded shoulders, soft features, and relatively youthful proportions of the torso to the head, the head being slightly larger than average relative to the body. Arms are shorter and hands and feet usually smaller than average.

It is important that you remember that even though we can with some justification make these kinds of groupings, each person is unique in her own balance of humors and in her particular manifestation of temperament. A choleric dominant man whose second humor was melancholic would differ in many ways from one whose second humor is sanguine. And two choleric gentlemen may still not appear as twins. Still, you and I and everyone has one dominant humor that can tell you a great deal about yourself and others without even getting into the details of the more subordinate humors. You will hear more about them when we explore ways to rebalance the humors.

Figure 2 compares in caricature the physical differences to which each humor tends, as summarized in Figure I.

Figure 3 describes the facial characteristics most often found associated with each humor and includes a typical manifestation of those characteristics. The sanguine dominant face tends to be

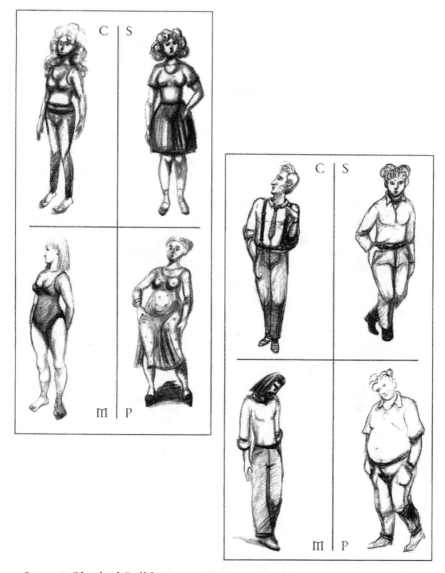

FIGURE 2. **Physical Build.** Here are four women and four men who are representatives of each of the four humoral temperaments, in their physical build and also their apparent demeanor and body language. Of course keep in mind that every person is completely individual, as are each of these people, so don't assume that all melancholics have straight hair or that all sanguines have curly. In assessing your humors, use the text to identify clusters of characteristics after you have gauged your first impression. No one will fit all the characteristic traits perfectly. Illustrations by Robert Rayevsky.

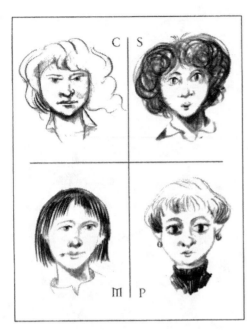

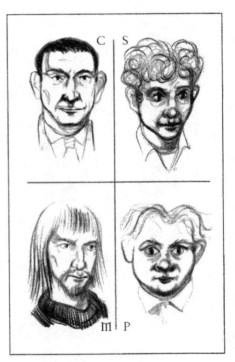

FIGURE 3. **Facial Qualities.** Here are four men and four women who are good representatives of the four humoral temperaments. Typically, the choleric face is squarish, brows are straight, mouth is straight, jaw is strong and square, eyes are close to nose, forehead is wide with a straight hairline. The sanguine face is heart shaped, with widow's peak for women, early hair recession from the center in men, small chin, deep-set almond eyes, narrowing forehead, small lips. The melancholic face is oval or oblong, with shallow-set eyes, arched eyebrows, high forehead, and full, wide lips, and recession at the temples in men. The phlegmatic face is rounded, large for the body, with rounded eyes and cheeks, and small mouth. Of course few have all the characteristic features. Look for the dominant cluster. Illustrations by Robert Rayevsky.

heart-shaped with deep-set, almond-shaped eyes and petite, rosebud mouth, and often curly hair. The melancholic dominant face tends to be oval in shape, with large eyes set shallowly, with a high forehead, wide mouth, full lips, and usually straight hair. The choleric dominant face is usually more square in shape, with wide, squared jaw and mouth, thin lips, eyes more close together, straight brows, and wavy hair. The phlegmatic face tends to be rounded, with small rounded eyes and childlike rounded cheeks, a petite mouth, and delicate hair.

Again, please keep in mind that these descriptions are in no way meant to typecast people in any negative way. There is no substitute for getting to know someone. But we are constantly picking up nonverbal and unconscious cues about ourselves and others. It makes sense then to use natural clusters of characteristics that can lead us more quickly to a deeper appreciation of preferences and possibilities in ourselves and the people we know and meet. You will learn more as we go on about how magnificently each person is equipped with his own unique gifts and how the humors can help you to find more direction and passion, cooperation, and companionship in your life.

Figure 4 gives you an idea of the hands of each prototypical humoral candidate. It is fun to examine the hands of an acquaintance old or new and see what you can tell about them. Then you can make conversation by asking questions to see if what you are guessing is true. The melancholic person with the long tapered fingers will usually say yes if you ask, "You would probably prefer a week of play and solitude in the breezy Caribbean to a week touring with a group and climbing in Alaska right?"

Skin varies with temperament. Choleric skin is more thick and coarse, while phlegmatic skin is youthful, supple, and thin. Melancholics have the most delicate skin, smooth and uniform in color when in perfect health. Sanguine skin tends toward pink, of medium thickness, relatively resilient, sensitive to sun.

Eyes vary significantly according to dominant humor. Sanguines have deep-set eyes while melancholics often have eyes that are shallow-set or even protruding. Cholerics have smaller

♠ C	S ♥
Large hands Squarish Large palm Solid fingers Firm grasp	Small hands Knuckles at base of fingers broad Fleshy palm Fingers short, thick Strong grasp
Narrow hands Long, tapered Classic for nail polish ads Slender fingers Gentle grasp	Small hands Delicate, rounded Rounded palm Small fingers Weak grasp
♦ ℍ	P ♣

FIGURE 4. **Telltale Hands.** Like face and body, the hands suggest an overriding tendency toward one or the other dominant humor in the temperament of each person. When in doubt because of variations in face and build, especially if your prospect is well clothed or extremely slight or heavy—hiding key features of bone structure and weight distribution—check the hands. Undoubtedly, experienced palm readers use their intuition with respect to these tendencies, whether they know the humors or not.

eyes, often a little closer together than melancholics or phlegmatics, perhaps more noticeably because of the broad jaw and
forehead. Phlegmatics have small eyes but rounded and spread
wide, giving a very open, childlike appearance.

Melancholics have large, even front teeth that remain fairly white.
Sanguines have smaller teeth than may be uneven and discolor more
easily. Cholerics have wide mouths of even teeth, and phlegmatics
often have quite small, sometimes crowded but fairly white teeth.

In men, sanguines have the most dramatic early development
of male-pattern baldness, while melancholics have recession at
the temples. Phlegmatics and cholerics are more prone to keep
their hair. Sad, isn't it? But if your humors are in balance, it
won't matter, because your hair will appear in perfect synchronicity with the wonderful person you are.

In women, the choleric usually has large breasts, the phlegmatic
the smallest. Sanguine breasts are perky, melancholic more bul-
bous. Cholerics and phlegmatics have more straight waistlines,
while melancholics and sanguines have the more cinched waistlines.
Just what you wanted to know! The good news is, that if your
humors are balanced, you will look absolutely wonderful because
you are your best you!

Melvin Page developed a very specific set of measurements of
the relative circumferences of different points on the forearms
and calves from which he could conclude the actual hormonal
balance of the person during her developmental years. We will
not get that specific here. You can find his work in the bibliography at the end of the book if you would like to learn more. You
can imagine my excitement when in studying his methods, I
found such strong contemporary validation for the four ancient
humoral prototypes. Other endocrinologists, such as Elliot
Abravanel, M.D., have described similar clusters of characteristics that match well with the humors and their temperaments.

The physical characteristics of each temperament are the least
important from the point of view of change, because you can't
change your basic physical structure. If you are over twenty, for
example, and you wish you had longer legs, bringing your humors
into balance will not change that. But these physical characteristics

are most important from the point of view of discovering you core humoral makeup.

Once you know your humoral tendencies, though, you can deeply affect your health, romance, and happiness for the better and your basic sense of self-esteem and appreciation for your own unique being. Most of the characteristics you will be looking at in the rest of the book, however, can be affected, corrected, and benefited by humoral awareness and rebalancing. Let's look at body fat accumulation, for example. Yes, there's some good news. It can be changed if you pay attention to your humors!

Most doctors and even exercise physiologists have said for decades that there is little that can be done to spot-reduce fat in specific areas of the body. But a whole industry of exercise machinery and personal trainers has grown up around the belief that it can be done. Is it possible?

The influence of the humors does cause different areas of the body to store fat at different rates. Often when the humors are brought into better balance in your body, through methods you will hear about in just a bit, fat deposits that have been resistant for years can disappear. And this, often without vigorous exercise! If you want to use exercise, the rebalancing may give you the energy and motivation to actually do the exercise you wish.

Figure 5 shows where each humor tends to deposit stored fat. The choleric will show the so-called male pattern, with little accumulated below the waist, but most showing up around the upper middle, shoulders, neck, and upper arms. In women these types become big bosomed and keep very narrow hips and legs.

The melancholic puts on weight in the breasts in women, in the belly, at the backs of the upper arms, and in the saddlebags or sides of the thighs, especially in women. In men it shows up mostly at the belly area, adding forward, not to the sides. Melancholic women maintain a waistline even after some weight gain.

The sanguine stores weight in the thighs, particularly the inner thighs and backs of thighs, and in the buttocks. Both men and women show a pear shape, though it's more dramatic with women. Sanguine women find very little change in their upper body, though they often would like to see an increase in bustline.

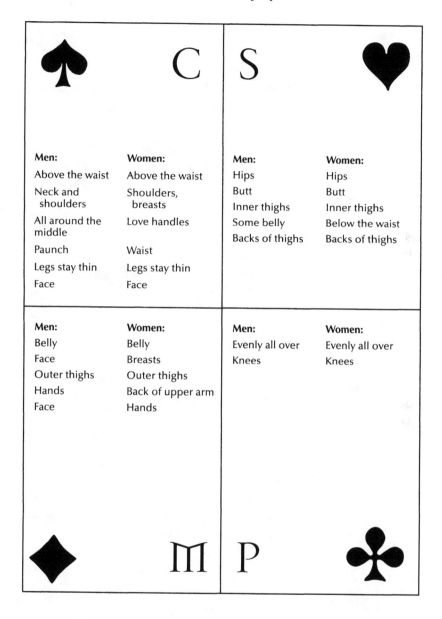

♠ C | S ♥

Men:
Above the waist
Neck and shoulders
All around the middle
Paunch
Legs stay thin
Face

Women:
Above the waist
Shoulders, breasts
Love handles
Waist
Legs stay thin
Face

Men:
Hips
Butt
Inner thighs
Some belly
Backs of thighs

Women:
Hips
Butt
Inner thighs
Below the waist
Backs of thighs

Men:
Belly
Face
Outer thighs
Hands
Face

Women:
Belly
Breasts
Outer thighs
Back of upper arm
Hands

Men:
Evenly all over
Knees

Women:
Evenly all over
Knees

♦ � P ♣

FIGURE 5. **Distribution of Weight Gain.** Fat added to the body tends to accumulate in characteristic places depending on the humor and temperament. People trying to lose weight may cut back in ways that pamper and indulge their dominant humor, and their unwanted fat will persist in all the wrong places. Instead, if they cut back on their craved foods and let their dominant humor rest, they are likely to lose where they want to lose and maintain where they want to maintain.

The phlegmatic person of either sex tends to add weight fairly evenly all over the body. These individuals often complain of chubby knees, while the other types accumulate little fat there. Their faces may get rounder, while the melancholics and sanguines in particular add little fat to the face. Arms too can get a little pudgy, to the phlegmatic's chagrin.

Cholerics and melancholics have a much easier time taking weight off than do the sanguines and phlegmatics. You will see how that comes about when you understand how each humor tends to burn fuel for energy.

Cholerics burn a lot of energy and can lose weight quickly. But also they can get large over time because they can develop huge appetites to accommodate their high level of activity. Melancholics are more sporadic dieters. They can lose quickly because of their intensity of life, but they often have trouble keeping it off unless they happen upon a dietary program that works for their sporadic energy levels. It depends on how they eat.

Phlegmatics have the hardest time losing weight, because of their slow energy burn, about which you'll find out more later. Sanguines produce energy very efficiently and also have a harder time losing weight. You will learn a whole lot more about achieving ideal weight and what's more important, your ideal figure, when you get to the section of the book that explores food preferences and dietary balance.

At this point, you might review the physical characteristics described here and compare how each of them may describe tendencies on your own part, referring back to your conclusions from the questionnaire in Chapter 2. Then think about some of the people you're close to among family and friends, or coworkers. See what clusters of qualities you can detect and what humors they represent. Do you notice how you have a bit more understanding and appreciation about who they are?

You might also consider what type of person sparks your romantic urges on first sight. You'll be learning more about this aspect of the humors before long when we turn to the phenomenon of attraction between temperaments.

For now you can find out more in the next chapter about the personality traits that tend to cluster with the physical traits you have just been exploring.

⁂

The human body contains blood, phlegm, yellow bile and black bile. These are the things that make up its constitution and cause its pains and health. Health is primarily that state in which these constituent substances are in the correct proportion to each other, both in strength and quantity, and are well mixed. Pain occurs when one of the substances presents either a deficiency or an excess, or is separated in the body and not mixed with the others. . . .

Common usage has assigned to them specific and different names because there are essential differences in their appearance. . . . They are different to the sense of touch. . . . They are dissimilar in their qualities of heat, cold, dryness and moisture. . . . If you give a man medicine which brings up phlegm, you will find his vomit is phlegm; if you give him one which brings up bile, he will vomit bile. Similarly, black bile can be eliminated by administering a medicine which brings it up, or, if you cut the body so as to form an open wound, it bleeds. When a drug is ingested, it first causes the evacuation of whatever in the body is naturally suited to it, but afterwards, it causes the voiding of other substances too. . . .

All these substances, then, are all always present in the body but vary in their relative quantities, each preponderating in turn according to its natural characteristics. . . . In the same way, if any of these primary bodily substances were absent from man, life would cease.

—HIPPOCRATES (c. 460-377 BCE), *The Nature of Man,*
in Lloyd, *Hippocratic Writings,* pp. 262–65

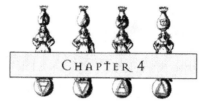

CHAPTER 4

Your Humoral Temperament:
Personality by the Humors

These four functional types correspond to the obvious means by which consciousness obtains its orientation to experience. *Sensation* (i.e., sense perception) tells you that something exists; *thinking* tells you what it is; *feeling* tells you whether it is agreeable or not; and *intuition* tells you whence it comes and where it is going.

The reader should understand that these four criteria of types of human behavior are just four viewpoints among many others, like will power, temperament, imagination, memory, and so on. There is nothing dogmatic about them, but their basic nature recommends them as suitable criteria for classification. I find them particularly helpful when I am called upon to explain parents to children and husbands to wives, and vice versa. They are also useful in understanding one's own prejudices.

—CARL G. JUNG (1875-1961), "Approaching the Unconscious,"
in Jung, *Man and His Symbols*, pp. 49–50

HE FOUR HUMORS are best known today for their psychological implications. Melancholy is a well-known mental state of sadness or depression. In fact, it is a major reason for the purchase of billions of dollars worth of antidepressant pharmaceutical drugs all over America. What if balancing the humors could change all that!

Phlegmatic is defined in psychological terms as lethargic, lacking in energy. We hear the word most often in describing cold symptoms. The phlegm of a cold certainly does slow you down. You will find out more about this when you read about the disease tendencies of the humors.

Sanguine is sometimes heard to refer to a mood that is optimistic, upbeat, pleasant, sometimes unreasonably so.

Choleric is probably the least frequently heard in everyday conversation, but it is still used occasionally to describe an angry overbearing kind of person, who's showing his "choler." Also "choler" is the Greek word for bile, and angry people are sometimes called bilious even today. Or we may hear, "He's showing his bile." This is a direct reference to the ancient humors as used in English since the days of Shakespeare.

In Jung's four ways of knowing in the opening quote above, we could say that the phlegmatic is most focused on the senses, the melancholic on thinking, the sanguine on feeling, and the choleric on intuition.

The Modern Masters
of the Humors

THE RENAISSANCE MASTERS of the humors were less focused on establishing the science and cosmology of the humors than were the ancients. They were more focused on the rich applications to character, satire, and cultural symbols. With the coming of modern medicine, advocates of the humoral school were relegated to the fringe, considered alternative, holistic, sometimes quacks. But today, as we move into the twenty-first century with groundbreaking new clinical research and applications, their prescience can be better appreciated.

WILLIAM SHAKESPEARE, 1564–1616

The most famous writer in the English language. He wrote dramas, histories, comedies, and tragedies. He performed in Ben Jonson's *Every Man in His Humour.* Made many references in his plays to the four humors and their impact on medicine and personality. It may not be going too far to suggest that his understanding of the full implications of the humors made his characters among the most realistic and memorable of all times and cultures. Four hundred years of Hamlet has left us with an unforgettable image of the melancholic, for example. Portia, the splendid master of argument in *The Merchant of Venice,* is a classic sanguine, believing in the essential good nature of humankind and being able to argue the point persuasively. Othello was the choleric leader among leaders, brought down by jealous deceivers who sparked his powerful anger and retribution. And so on.

BEN JONSON, 1572–1637

English dramatist and satirist of social pretensions, author of *Every Man in His Humour* (first performed in 1598) and *Every Man Out of His Humour* (1599). He used the humors in his later plays as well and played repeatedly with the question whether in any situation they applied to physiology, psychology, social pretensions, or all three. His works made the temperaments and their rich vocabulary a permanent part of the English language, being all the rage once again in Victorian England.

Emanuel Swedenborg, 1688–1772

Swedish mystic, theologian, and scientist. He inspired the Swedenborgian Church, which was based on his mystical experiences after 1743. Wrote works on philosophy, metaphysics, metallurgy, anatomy, and physiology, as well as thirty volumes on his religious revelations. He developed a complex system of correspondences related to ancient alchemy and rich with religious symbolism. Like Paracelsus, he knew much about metal but became more interested in the "metal" of the spirit. Among his many followers are the poet William Blake, evangelist Johnny Appleseed, and writer Helen Keller.

Thomas Sydenham, 1624–1689

English physician, called "the English Hippocrates." He was author of *Observationes Medicae* and like Hippocrates advocated careful observation, rather than theory, in treating patients. Similarly, he pre-scribed simple lifestyle changes such as fresh air and horseback rid-ing, rather than more invasive measures, always responding to the need to rebalance the humors.

Samuel Hahnemann, 1755-1843

German physician and founder of homeopathy, based on his dis-covery that infinitesimally small amounts of substances tended to create in healthy people the same symptoms that they cured in sick people. It's the idea of "the hair of the dog that bit you" as a remedy for dog bite. He was well versed in the works of Avicenna and other traditional physicians, and geared his controversial remedies to the specific constitutional types or temperaments of his patients. He considered psychological symptoms as telling as physical ones in determining the proper remedy for each patient. The practice of home-opathy has been growing steadily in Europe and achieved recent popu-larity in the United States as patients have begun to question the powerful medications offered by conventional modern medicine, with their dangerous ancillary effects and sometimes dubious or addictive results.

Rudolf Steiner, 1861–1925

Austrian social philosopher, theosophist, founder of anthroposophy. An expert on the German poet and dramatist Goethe, he emphasized the importance of spiritual perception, especially in education and therapy. His work inspired some seventy Rudolf Steiner Schools, still operating. He wrote *Occult Science: An Outline* (1913), and *Knowledge of the Higher Worlds and Its Attainment,* among other works. His system of healing is based on rebalancing the four humors, and his program for education is based on the sequential development of body, mind, spirit, and soul.

Carl Gustav Jung, 1875–1961

Swiss psychiatrist, leading collaborator with Sigmund Freud from 1907 to 1913. He developed the idea of psychological "complexes," the "collective unconscious," "introvert and extrovert," and four archetypes of our basic nature. In his foreword to the English edition of Jolande Jacobi's *Paracelsus: Selected Writings* (1941), Jung describes Paracelsus as "a preoccupation of mine when I was trying to understand alchemy, especially its connection to natural philosophy." He wrote *Psychology and Alchemy* (1944), and was one of the giants of the twentieth century for his influence on modern psychology, particularly for the idea of an essential drive to the spiritual in each of us, for the idea of a balance of male and female in each, and for the four archetypes, which now are considered basic to most psychological classifications and testing, whether of a popular or academic nature. The latter are the sensing extrovert, who perceives primarily through the senses, the intuitive extrovert, who perceives intuitively, the sensing introvert, and the intuitive introvert. (These correspond to the melancholic, the choleric, the phlegmatic, and the sanguine, respectively.)

R. Swinburne Clymer, 1878–1966

American medical doctor and minister in the Church of Illumination. Published over one hundred works on philosophy, medicine, health, nutrition, and the occult, including *The Occult Compendium* and *The Mysteries of Osiris or Ancient Egyptian Initiation* (1951). He balanced a very practical approach to holistic nutrition from basic, quality foods with a spiritual and mystical aspect. He studied Paracelsus' work in detail and used it in his practice. He inspired the founding of the Clymer Clinic in Quakertown, Pennsylvania, which has inspired a number of the leading holistic doctors and health practitioners in the eastern United States.

Henry Bieler, contemporary

American physician, M.D., and nutritionist. Developed profiles for three endocrine types—adrenal, thyroid, and pituitary—and described their physical and personality characteristics. He recommended specific dietary support for each. He wrote *Food Is Your Best Medicine,* echoing the aphorism attributed to Hippocrates, "Let your food be your medicine and your medicine be your food."

Rudolf Hauschka, contemporary

German medical doctor, interpreter of Rudolf Steiner's work. Author of *Nutrition* (1951), *The Nature of Substance,* and other books on health. He uses the humors in his anthroposophic practice of healing and temperamental rebalancing.

Melvin E. Page, contemporary

American dentist, D.D.S., author on physical types and development, endocrinology, and nutrition. He found four general patterns, two sympathetic dominant and two parasympathetic dominant. Developed a system of measurements for guidance on the endocrine balance of his patients and used glandular extracts and nutrition to rebalance the body. He wrote *Degeneration—Regeneration,* describing his research.

Elliot D. Abravanel, contemporary

American physician, M.D., specializing in endocrinology. Author of books analyzing endocrine types, their physiological and psychological traits, and nutritional and lifestyle choices for each, for healthy weight loss and overall well-being. Author of *The Body Type Diet* and other contemporary popular works.

Kenneth Fordham, contemporary

American dentist, D.D.S., medical school professor, founder and director of the Fordham-Page Clinic for over thirty years, continuing the work of Melvin Page, especially with respect to sound nutrition and the four glandular types, which correspond well, as this book asserts, to the ancient typology of the temperaments and their humors.

Hakim G.M. Chishti, contemporary

American naturopathic doctor, N.D., interpreter of Avicenna's work, author of *The Traditional Healer's Handbook: A Classic Guide to the Medicine of Avicenna*. His work is an excellent resource on the temperaments in detail and the work of the famous Arabic and Muslim physician.

Robert Jenkins, contemporary

Doctor of chiropractic, D.C., and certified nutritionist. Founder of the Clymer Clinic and inspired by Dr. Clymer's work, he is a student of Paracelsus' work on spiritual alchemy and a member of the Paracelsus Society.

The famous Swiss psychologist Carl G. Jung went into great detail in analyzing the four temperaments or personality types, what he called "archetypes," in all different dimensions. His work has been so elaborated that some typological schemes for personality, based on his work, have up to sixty-four different categories based on how you process information, whether you are introverted or extroverted, and so on. One major example is the Myers-Briggs classification system used in many career counseling and employment situations. You do not need that much detail to appreciate and use the concept of the humors in your daily life, but check the Bibliography if you want to learn more about these.

Jung was, in turn, a serious investigator of the writings of Paracelsus, the enigmatic theologian, philosopher, and doctor of the early sixteenth century who was a master at using and interpreting the humors. Jung was sufficiently impressed with their relevance, it seems, to have used them as a foundation for his own groundbreaking work in modern psychoanalysis and therapy. His "collective unconscious" may have a lot to do with the intuitive knowledge we are investigating in this book about how our human characteristics tend to cluster across populations.

Let's look now at some of the most ancient associations as they touch on personality.

The choleric humor corresponds to fire. It is bright like the sun. The choleric woman or man is a person of vision and intuition. She makes decisions with a laser-like assessment and definitive answer, from the gut, with total confidence. She is slow to anger because few things can distract her from her goal, but her anger is swift and decisive if it erupts. She has no time for ambiguity. She can burn you up in her forward motion without even realizing it. She is a person of action—she gets things done. She feels a strong responsibility of leadership and competes aggressively to be the best. She likes to see things to comprehend them and grasps ideas quickly.

The phlegmatic humor corresponds to water. It flows. The phlegmatic man does whatever needs to be done. He takes hold of tasks and completes them reliably and consistently. Even the most tedious work gives him satisfaction when it is done well. He learns crafts and skills quickly, carefully, and masterfully. Dedication, devotion, and helping people or a cause have great value to him. Loyalty and family are deep motivations. Solutions to problems through attention to detail and group effort give him great pride. He angers easily but forgives easily. He loves to relax after work, laugh, and play with family and friends. He is friendly, cheerful, sometimes shy. He is flexible, very accepting of those around him, but immovable when basic values are at stake.

The melancholic humor corresponds to the earth. It is the most grounded of the humors. The melancholic woman or man can vary tremendously from being very earthy in language or humor or dress to being flighty, mobile, and highly poetic and expressive. Nature has huge impact on the melancholic. She is much like mercury, one of the thickest liquid elements, that goes up and down dramatically with the atmospheric pressure. Melancholics are in fact very sensitive to weather changes. She can swing from very playful and social to withdrawn and solitary. She can anger very quickly and will often hold on to a grudge for some time. She makes decisions either on a whim or very deliberately, and either way can doubt her decisions later because of her changeability and her fervent desire to be grounded in the truth.

The most famous melancholic in all of literature would be Shakespeare's Hamlet. He is passionate, changeable, a superb actor, self-deprecating, creative, quick-witted, artistic, and athletic. He is also haunted by skepticism, indecision, melancholy, a desire to escape, and mercurial highs and lows. In her book *Hamlet's Choice*, Linda Kay Hoff writes, "Re the cause of Hamlet's delay, theories range from Stoll's succinct *plus de piece possible*, to Schlegel's action inhibiting skepticism, to melancholy as the factotum of Elizabethan abnormal psychology, to Nietzsche's nausea."

The sanguine humor corresponds to the air. It is the humor of communication, passion, relatedness. It is sometimes called wind or breath, since air as a substance was not even known until several hundred years ago. But the ancients knew that the blood was very responsive to the breath. The sanguine man can be accused of being a windbag, or full of hot air, because he or she is so driven to talk, persuade, interact, communicate. He angers slowly and forgives quickly, because he craves relationships. He makes decisions based on the effects on all present and rarely reconsiders. He loves promoting get-togethers and attending events and is often one of the last to leave. He likes meeting new people and seldom feels the need to be alone.

To summarize personalities, one might describe the choleric temperament as "driven," the phlegmatic as "kind," the melancholic as "intense," and the sanguine as "clever."

Figures 6 and 7 describe some typical characteristics of the way each humoral type responds to anger and to joy. Figures 8 and 9 delineate some of the different ways the dominant humors show themselves depending on whether the person's humors are in or out of balance.

As you can see from Figure 8, each humor has its own cluster of unpleasant characteristics that arise when the humors are out of balance. The best qualities of each humor become their worst when the humors are out of balance or in disharmony. If your dominant humor is either diminished or excessive, for example, by neglect or overstimulation, respectively, then the worst traits of temperament arise. You might be called "temperamental" by way of criticism.

That's when the choleric's decisive leadership can turn aggressive and oppressive. The sanguine's gift for relating to people can turn into argumentation, sarcasm, and pleading. The phlegmatic's loyalty and trusting nature makes him vulnerable to a sense of betrayal and desire for rebellion and change for change's sake. The melancholic's playful flexibility can become serious unreliability.

As you will hear soon, clear steps can be taken in each case to restore balance. Instead of combating directly the unpleasant or even debilitating mood, or God forbid, medicating it with powerful drugs that mask or suppress it, other avenues become suddenly obvious with awareness of the temperaments, to help reinforce or soften a humor. This is so, you will see later, because the humors share a broad band of correspondences with various environmental and other conditions that we can control and

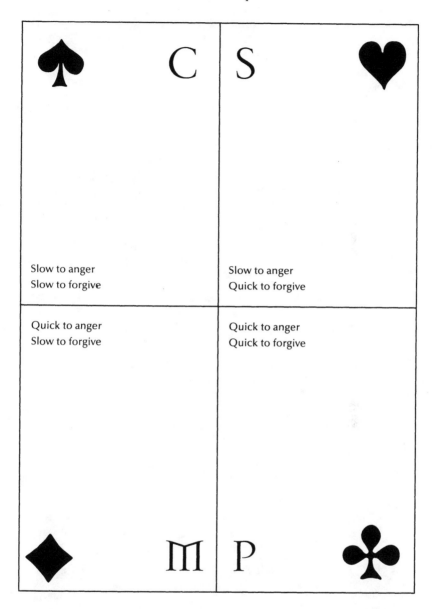

FIGURE 6. Expressing Anger. Each temperament has a characteristic expression of anger. You may notice that the temperaments diagonal to each other might be considered complementary opposites. The choleric does not ruffle easily but once crossed, never forgets. The phlegmatic notices affronts quickly but also gets over them fast. The melancholic angers easily but may not let you know it and may hold on to a grudge. The sanguine has a high tolerance for offense but after talking it out forgives promptly.

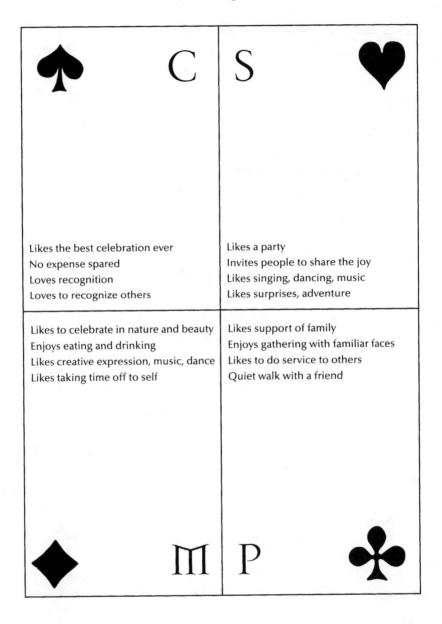

♠ C	S ♥
Likes the best celebration ever No expense spared Loves recognition Loves to recognize others	Likes a party Invites people to share the joy Likes singing, dancing, music Likes surprises, adventure
Likes to celebrate in nature and beauty Enjoys eating and drinking Likes creative expression, music, dance Likes taking time off to self	Likes support of family Enjoys gathering with familiar faces Likes to do service to others Quiet walk with a friend
♦ Ⅲ	P ♣

FIGURE 7. Expressing Joy. The temperaments tend toward different modes of expression for positive emotions. Diagonals may be complementary. People of a particular temperament can feel vaguely unsatisfied after a happy event if they do not experience their own way of being joyful.

♠ C	S ♥
Domineering	Argumentative
Aggressive	Bombastic
Condescending	Self-blaming
Insistent	Weepy
Overbearing	Obstinate
Mercurial	Impulsive
Withdrawn	Rebellious
Accusatory	Lethargic
Defensive	Crying
Anxious	Complaining
♦ Ⅲ	P ♣

FIGURE 8. **Symptoms of Imbalance.** Each temperament has a characteristic cluster of behaviors that appear when the person is out of balance—in bad humor. That is, when the dominant humor is either in excess or depletion. It can help to learn these profiles and recognize them if you imagine their connection to the elements associated with each humor. For example, the choleric can behave forcefully like fire, while the sanguine can be "full of hot air," the melancholic can be heavy like the earth, and the phlegmatic can be tearful and reactive, like water.

♠ C	S ♥
Magnanimous	Wise
Inspiring	Empathetic
Enrolling	Encouraging
Charismatic	Trusting
Visionary	Communicative
Intuitive	Humorous
Decisive	Compassionate
Creative	Masterful
Enthusiastic	Steadfast
Playful	Supportive
Insightful	Faithful
Analytical	Persistent
Galvanizing	Loyal
Imaginative	Skilled
♦ ♏	P ♣

FIGURE 9. **Signs of Good Balance.** When people are in good humor, the best of their temperaments shine through, but with flexibility and grace so their characteristic traits are not exaggerated into faults. Like fire, the choleric can light up a room and ignite a great enterprise. Like air, the sanguine can move easily from one person to another and create better communication and understanding. Like earth, the melancholic can create new life in others and make things grow. Like water, the phlegmatic can nurture and nourish and move mountains with quiet persistence.

change subtly and safely to achieve healthy changes in the humors. This way, the body's wisdom is not short-circuited but is allowed instead to achieve its natural, vibrant balance.

You will hear more about these remedial measures later. But first what many have been waiting for—the implications for romance and other relationships.

Swedenborg proposed that correspondences operate through built-in channels within the psyche, which react to our perceptions of the physical world. Every aspect of creation—sun and stars, earth and air, fire and water, minerals and plants, birds, beasts, creeping things, and other people—each of these triggers a specific resonance somewhere deep within us, beneath the surface of ordinary awareness.

—HARVEY BELLIN, "'Opposition is True Friendship,'
Swedenborg's Influences on William Blake,"
in Larsen, *Emanuel Swedenborg, A Continuing Vision* (1988), p. 97

CHAPTER 5

Your Humoral Relationships:
Romance and Friends by the Humors

And so there is and should be only one love between a man and a woman and no other.

But the love of the man compared to a woman's is in its heat like the fire of burning mountains, which is difficult to put out—compared to a fire of wood which is easily extinguished. And the love of the woman compared to the love of the man is like the gentle heat of the sun which produces fruit, compared to a fiercely blazing fire of wood, since she gently offers her fruit in offspring. But the great love that was in Adam, when Eve was taken from him, and the sweetness of that slumber in which he was sleeping were turned to a contrary mode of sweetness by his transgression.

—HILDEGARD OF BINGEN (1098–1179), "Causes and Cures,"
in Flanagan, *Secrets of God: Writings of Hildegard of Bingen,* p. 113

ATER AND FIRE are drawn together, while air and earth have a mutual attraction. If this is not immediately obvious to you, that's okay! We cannot here go into all the esoteric thinking about the interaction of elements that ancient philosophers like Aristotle and others indulged in to try to explain the universe. It is enough perhaps to say that the universe was viewed as composed of four strata, earth below, then the oceans around the earth, then the air above the earth and then the fire above that, including the sun, lightning, and the stars, which all gave off their light by burning. The ancients linked the earth and ocean with the female aspects of creation, and the air and fire with the male aspects of creation.

Certainly in any particular gendered person there are elements of both male and female aspects of creation. But in a broadbrush sort of way, virtually every traditional society on earth has made the same sort of linkage as the ancient Greeks did when they developed the humors to their finest art. This ubiquitous linkage probably goes back to the fact that the female reproductive cycle is obviously linked to the moon, as are the tides of the ocean. This leaves the sun, the moon's counterpart by day, for the male. Women do much of their most important work by the light of the moon, gathering herbs and suckling sleepy children. Also their reproductive force is hidden inside the body, compact and mysterious like the earth and the ocean and night itself.

In contrast, the male reproductive cycle responds to the sun, the yearly cycle, with more activity in the long days of summer. Likewise many male activities in a traditional society occur during daylight. Building, hunting, herding. Also, their reproductive force is outside the body, obvious, visible, forceful, like wind and sun.

All this is to say that the humors of choler and sanguine are most identified with the male aspect of creativity and the melancholic and phlegm with the female aspect. In the analysis of character, this tends to mean that the choleric and sanguine tend to be more assertive and proactive influences among the humors, while the melancholic and phlegmatic are the more private and responsive humoral influences.

In general, the choleric humor and the sanguine humor tend to be romantically attracted to the phlegmatic and melancholic respectively, the more male elements being attracted to the more female elements. This does not imply for a minute that a melancholic man is any less manly than a choleric man or a sanguine woman any less womanly than a phlegmatic. We are talking only about esoteric associations that seem to lead to some helpful practical predictions when applied in different situations. What in fact happens is that different elements of manliness and womanliness will tend to show up depending on the balance of humors in the particular man or woman.

Not too many today will claim women can't be just as assertive as men, or any man as receptive or responsive as any woman. But all in all, a sanguine or choleric woman will definitely tend to be more assertive than a melancholic or phlegmatic woman. And a melancholic or phlegmatic man will tend in general to be more reflective and responsive than a sanguine or choleric man when he is in his humor.

For this very reason, the ancient humoral way of understanding human attractions should not be limited by any presumptions about the physical genders of any particular romantic partners. Though traditionally texts refer to male/female pairings for a number of reasons, it is well known that in every society throughout human history same-sex attractions have played an important role in human relations and have been the basis of a significant minority of romantic relationships. Be encouraged then not to limit the power of the insights offered here by assuming they might not apply to any particular relationship.

Duality and the Humors

THE CREATION STORIES of ancient civilizations around the world have attributed the origin of the universe to the creation of a duality out of nothingness. The ancient Chinese tradition of Lao Tzu, for example, contrasted yin and yang—the cool, dark, contracting energy and the bright, warm, expanding energy.

The ancient Hebrews described God creating light and darkness, heaven and earth, Adam and Eve. Native Americans describe their heritage, and future, as a balance and interaction between the father sun and the mother earth. And early twentieth century psychoanalyst Wilhelm Reich postulated that a pulsation between contraction and expansion—between female and male—was the key to understanding all of existence.

Today, quantum physicists speculate about how the world emerged from a homogenous vacuum into a diverse universe comprised of a duality of matter and anti-matter.

When the ancient Greeks developed the four humors, they identified them with this universal duality. The choleric and sanguine were warmer, more active, more concentrated, and more expansive substances. They gave rise to classically male qualities, like focus, assertiveness, power, and passion. The melancholic and phlegmatic were cooler, slower, more dispersed and more contracting substances. They gave rise to classically female qualities, like attentiveness, responsiveness, patience, and devotion.

Meanwhile, the choleric represented the drier, more aggressive and intuitive kind of male energy and the sanguine represented the more diluted, more deliberate and circumspect kind of male energy. The melancholic brought out the drier, more independent style of female energy, while the phlegmatic represented the more tender, nurturing style of female energy.

Any assumptions about gender links to activities or attitudes can be highly provocative today and must come under strict scrutiny. But to try to eliminate the ancient associations or deny them some validity may be like throwing the baby out with the bath water. It is hard to deny, for example, that a nurturing, attentive mother and a strong, protective father are not key contributors to the success of a human child and indeed to the survival and success of a human tribe, society, and indeed the species. So instead, consider how proper use of the humors can help deal with current issues and avoid oversimplifications and stereotypes in at least two important ways.

First, since every one of us has all four humors, we cannot draw any conclusions about how people will behave—whether groups of men or groups of women or any particular man or woman—based purely on gender. Your temperament takes its character from the humor which dominates when a stress causes the need for energy and adjustment. But all humors are always present, whether blocked, diminished, excessive, or in dynamic equilibrium. This means that both male and female tendencies exist in all people.

To illustrate, in our current world of abbreviated words and images, we may assume that if we say male energy is more bold and aggressive while female energy is more patient and enduring, then a "real" man must be bold and aggressive and a "real" woman must be patient and enduring. In fact, every individual has his or her own dynamic balance of these energies.

Secondly, the duality of male and female energies is a powerful tool for understanding creativity and avoiding simplistic judgments about the relative value of various activities and roles in society. The creative process encompasses the full range of human activity, including the creation and nurturing of children by a man and a woman, the love in all human bonding, personal growth and transformation, and self-expression in art or action. The ancient traditions hold that both female and male energies must be present for creativity, just as sperm and egg must be present to conceive, and right and left brain must interact for meaningful thought. Duality explains not only past creation but also creation ongoing, as it moves the present forward.

For illustration, consider recent shifts in society. Twenty years ago, educated women wanted to liberate themselves from domestic enslavement through academic achievement and employment in the market place. The economy was transformed and the roles inside the home became much more fluid and often controversial. But lately, many educated women are choosing to put a high value on full time parenting and home making, postponing careers and degrees. The difference is choice and self value.

The four humors and the temperaments can bring these into focus.

All this is leading up to the interesting result that cholerics and phlegmatics attract each other, and melancholics and sanguines attract each other. Opposites do attract.

This does not necessarily mean disharmony is inevitable. Quite the contrary. The choleric and phlegmatic are both interested in strength and loyalty, the choleric from the leadership end and the phlegmatic from the support and mastery end. They are opposites in many ways but these core values draw them together and they intuit a special complementarity between them.

Likewise, the melancholic and sanguine share an interest in passion and adventure, the melancholic from the natural and earthy end of the spectrum and the sanguine from the human relational and cosmic end of the same spectrum.

It is fun to notice how many marriages that have withstood the test of time, not just five years but twenty-five years or more, exhibit this kind of humoral attraction and complementarity.

This also explains the often befuddling phenomenon of people who look so different physically being gaga for each other. Often a tall willowy woman will fall in love with a short balding man, and people will wonder why. But their temperaments match. She is likely to be melancholic dominant with a tendency to be moody and perhaps disorganized and maybe unsure of herself. She is drawn to his sanguine temperament, steady and ready to communicate anytime, often with a sense of humor that brightens her mood. He tends to be organized in his life and flattering to her by his attention and consistency.

A dramatic example of such a pair appears in the 1988 film *Who Framed Roger Rabbit?* A bumbling cartoon rabbit named Roger has the undying affection of a tall, glamorous human cartoon woman named Jessica. People marvel at how she who could have anyone is totally devoted to him. She says, "Because he makes me laugh." A great melancholic/sanguine pair!

The sexual appetites associated with the humors can be of particular interest to committed partners, since complementary partners have different inclinations for how often they want to get together. Imagine if by balancing the humors, with a small change in diet, for example, you could bring a couple back into the same ballpark in their desire for sex. This was exactly the case with one of the first couples I counseled using the humors.

You may remember Sharon and Gabe from the Introduction, with different tastes in food and different desires as far as frequency of sex. They were a phlegmatic wife and a sanguine husband. She consumed dairy, which accentuated her phlegmatic tendencies, including a relatively weak libido. Sex every week or two was more than enough for her. She was busy with kids and household and school and felt no need for more.

He indulged the sanguine taste for spicy foods, which emphasized his sanguine tendency toward a strong libido. He was ready at least once a day for some romance. He thought about it a lot and felt frustrated that her interest was so infrequent.

No more Szechuan or hot peppers for lunch at work for him. Less snacking and dieting on yogurt and cottage cheese for her. When each toned down those eating habits, which overstimulated their dominant humors, their sexual resentments diminished and their sexual interest mellowed in the direction of the other, so that their sex life improved dramatically! Rather than both appearing "temperamental" to each other, their temperaments matched.

In the 1977 film *Annie Hall*, Woody Allen's character tells his psychiatrist that they engage in sex almost never, only about three times a week. Diane Keaton's character, Annie, tells her psychiatrist that they have sex all the time, sometimes as much as three times a week. She is a classic melancholic, languid and beautiful, mildly depressed and self-absorbed. He is a classic sanguine, obsessed with relationships, witty and communicative, appearing cynical but willing to believe any problem can be solved. A classic sanguine and melancholic pair whose humors are sadly, but "humorously," exaggerated. Like another playwright, Shakespeare, Woody Allen had a fine grasp, whether he knew it or not, of humoral character and what happens to people when their humors are exaggerated by lifestyle and circumstance.

The choleric has a moderately strong libido, as does the melancholic. But the first is inclined to very regular experience, while the second goes in fits and starts, being eager for a few days and then off for a few. This is nice to know if you are married to someone with a melancholic temperament. Otherwise you might take it personally when your spouse's interest waxes and wanes in the course of a week. You might blame yourself without cause.

All this does not mean that a marriage cannot last if it is not between these two classic pairs—choleric/phlegmatic and melancholic/sanguine—but understanding the humors sure could be helpful in any such marriage. Imagine for example, a good-looking couple, both tall, exhibiting what is valued most by Western European fashion standards—tall, oval face, small boned, tapered limbs. What happens when they both get into a melancholic mood at the same time? In Hollywood they get divorced. But not everyone has that out. And there may be a better way.

While they are both indulging their mood, say one sips wine and the other downs cartons of ice cream or increases his running schedule, there will be no communication, virtually none. And most likely, each will blame the other and feel unloved.

It would be very helpful, you might imagine, to know that they just happened, both of them, to hit the bottom of their mercury at the same time. They need to know that if they just ride it out without hurting each other too much and rebalance their humors for themselves in their own favorite, constructive ways, then one or both will come out of it and the relationship can resume.

So don't worry if you are not married to or in relationship with someone of your complementary temperament. A lot more than temperament goes into who we pick as our life partners. But knowledge of your respective temperaments can help assure that your experience together is a good one.

If you are getting along, you have already discovered how to enrich your humor patterns to form a complementarity that pleases each of you. You can continue to do that with greater assurance and less experimentation now that you understand the humors.

If you have some stress in your relationship, the humors are a great tool for understanding where the gaps are in making the relationship more enjoyable and meaningful for both.

There is nothing that says your soul mate must be your direct opposite in humoral pattern. This is simply a tendency when it comes to attracting a partner. Many very successful couples are not direct opposites or may have the same humoral dominance. I will suggest, however, that they are successful because they have found ways to keep themselves in balance so that they are at their best for each other. Two melancholics at their worst will both withdraw into depression and quit. Two cholerics out of balance will try to dominate each other. Two sanguines will argue incessantly. Two phlegmatics out of balance will feel lost and confused and fall apart. But as a team of like-minded healthy people, any of these couples can succeed magnificently. Another good reason to know how to balance your humors!

Do you think it might be helpful to you if you have not found a life partner yet and are looking for one, to know ahead of time what kind of moods, sexual appetite, anger, expressions, fights, and forms of fun your prospect may be prone to, especially over a lifetime?

If you are a woman and you seem always to hook up with men who appear to be the life of the party and all attentiveness toward you, and then a week later are withdrawn and unavailable emotionally, you can actually decide, before you get too involved, whether you have the confidence and patience to put up with that melancholic, mercurial character.

Or if you are a man and you are drawn to sassy little ladies with tiny waists and engaging wit, are you ready for her sanguine tendency to organize you, to talk like there's no tomorrow to get a point across, to argue you under the table if you're wrong, and to feel hurt if you don't want to make love just about every day?

If the rugged bear-type fellow turns you on, are you prepared for his choleric tendency to be domineering when he is tired or frustrated in achieving his great visions, or can you handle his temptation to put some great cause or career ahead of family time?

If you are attracted to the perky, adorable woman whose age is impossible to tell and who laughs and twinkles like a teenager, are you ready for her phlegmatic tendency to act out in response to petty offenses and to be cautious one minute and impulsive the next?

Vibrational Health and the Humors

THERE MAY BE an apparent conflict here. On the one hand, we hear that opposites attract. On the other hand, we hear that like attracts like. Is there one rule for romance and another for friends? Or is the rule of opposites applicable to relationships while the rule of like applies to aspects of thought?

These ideas are not in essential conflict. They are in fact complementary. Today's success gurus and proponents of positive thinking say we become what we think about. They say that in the world of mind and spirit, we attract what we expect to attract. If we think negative thoughts, trouble comes. If we expect goodness in our lives, it is more likely to come.

Then why if a phlegmatic person is thinking about family and togetherness will she attract someone who is a choleric, all about forging out into the world and reaching pinnacles of community leadership? These roles are complementary in the plane of security and loyalty. The family-focused phlegmatic person who is in good humor "thinks" about security because she needs it to achieve a safe family, and the protector champion type can give it to her. Likewise, the champion-type choleric who is in good humor "thinks" about who needs protection and attracts that person.

If these two are on the same plane, knowing themselves and their desires and being open to complementarity and fulfillment, then each will be attracted to the other. They are attracting like to like, because both are in a healthy level of vibration.

Physics teaches us that everything, even all that we can touch and smell, is characterized most accurately by its vibrational profile. And two things will tend to come into synchronicity over time. Particles under experimental circumstances act like waves, not distinct particles. It is impossible to explore this concept very much further here, but much cutting-edge exploration of health and healing focuses on the levels of vibration of the body and mind. In the tissues, exciting medical research is showing that every organ has its own pitch and resonance. The healthier the organ is, the clearer and more harmonious its vibration with its surroundings. What's more, ailing organs can be made to return to health by application of specific fields of vibration that match the organ's ideal state. Likewise, it has been found that placing the body in a general magnetic field that simulates the natural vibration levels of the earth, which itself is a giant magnet, creates an environment in which organs can more easily reestablish their own healthy level of vibration.

Similarly, the power of prayer, and nonlocal thoughts directed to others, whether by caring family members, doctor, shaman, church congregation, or unidentified well-wishers, suggest that we are all connected by levels of vibration.

Building on the work of Carl G. Jung, who suggested a collective unconscious of mind/spirit, Larry Dossey, M.D., in his book *Reinventing Medicine,* quotes philosopher Michael Grosso for the proposition that the brain responds to mind as radios do to radio waves. Mind preexists outside the individual as a form of vibration, while the brain simply taps into the vibrations at will.

Shamanic medicine and the power of music, song, drumming, and laughter to heal are other avenues of exploration for the concept that health is essentially a quality of vibration, harmonious and clear. Chinese medicine, to mention just one more example, uses voice quality as a diagnostic tool. The idea of vibrational health shows up daily in our culture without our awareness. Just as "humor" entered the English common language in the sixteenth century, so vibrational vocabulary is part of our post-quantum language. For example, we speak of being "up to speed," "on the same wavelength," "turning up the amplitude," "being at the same frequency," "giving out good vibes" or "bad vibes," and "tuning in" or "tuning out."

Wilhelm Reich, controversial psychotherapist and colleague of Freud's, developed a cosmology of widespread pulsation, or vibration, which he explored in his book *The Function of Orgasm.*

These observations may give us reason to believe that the more similar a pair is in their level of vibrational health, the more attracted they will be to each other. A harmony is heard and felt between them. For example, a balanced sanguine, at a high level of vibration, that is, mind and body resonating in harmony, will not be attracted to a melancholic person who is out of balance, radiating dissonance, at a low level of vibration, emitting a disharmonious message from the plane of his life. But if the melancholic gets back into balance, gets back a "sense of humor," the attraction will be there.

It may be helpful to think for a moment about the humors in three dimensions. The dimension left to right is receptive to active. The dimension back to forward is physical focus to relational focus, or competitive focus to cooperative focus. And the dimension top to bottom is high level of humoral integrity to low level of humoral integrity. Trying to match up the eight different pairs now possible becomes a challenge, a bit like Rubik's Cube or three-dimensional tic-tac-toe. But consider how the out-of-balance melancholic may actually be more attracted to an out-of-balance choleric than to the healthy sanguine, since together they have fast metabolisms and like to eat under stress. Together they could dream (the melancholic) and plot (the choleric) revenge for their hardships. If one moves into the higher vibrational level, though, the attraction will vanish.

In a similar vein, the bad-tempered melancholic can easily fall for an out-of-temper sanguine, because the argumentative sanguine will give him lots of reasons to pass the blame for his problems on to others outside himself.

The bottom line here is that if you seek complementary harmonious relationships, don't spend a lot of time looking. Simply take steps to make yourself more attractive by raising your own level of vibration and using your own good sense of humor to maximize your temperamental health.

If you grasp the impact of the humors, you can certainly feel more in control if these things arise in your relationships. If you know your own humoral tendency to react, you can make a choice, too, about how far you will go in indulging the downside of your dominant humor. You can take steps to minimize your discomfort in any situation. And beyond that, you can make subtle changes in your living environment that can have a profound effect on you and on your partner's humoral balance.

For example, suppose your choleric wife is getting hot under the collar. Nothing pleases her and she starts ordering people around, including you. Check the environmental conditions. Chances are that conditions are just too hot and dry for her. Suggest a swim or a cool shower together, or simply a tall glass of ice water and all may be well. Or turn on the air-conditioning and buy her a thirty-dollar fountain for the living room table.

But more about comfort later.

The humors play a huge part in illuminating friendships too. Often Mutt and Jeff, or Oscar and Felix, are the rule rather than the exception. Observers may expect people who are alike to want to hang out together, but that's not really the way it works. The elements attract different elements to themselves. We hear that like attracts like, but this is a vibrational rule, not a material rule. If you are at a high vibration of health in your humors, you will tend to attract someone who is also at a high vibration of health. And if you are at an unhealthy, low vibrational extreme, you will attract someone else who is similarly suffering. But in each case, your partner will tend to be of a complementary humor.

Often we will find a great deal in common with a person and then wonder why we don't actually choose to spend a lot of time with them. It's because we don't want more of our already dominant humor. We seek complementarity.

One error that's easy to make in relationships is based on this desire for a difference, a challenge, something interesting to grow with in our relationship. We are seeking a healthy complementarity of humors. But since most people don't know this, they are mistakenly attracted to difficult people, who eat up their time and emotion merely by being difficult. As you gain an understanding of the humors, you will find your desire for adventure or growth or interest is better nurtured by someone whose humors are balanced and complementary to yours. Hold off on the difficult people until they have their humors in balance!

I remember in the 1970s, when the first computers were touted as being able to match up characteristics by huge databases. It seemed an awesome way to find a compatible date. But it didn't really catch on. We don't want people just like us. Today's automated dating analysis services ask you what you are looking for and match you up that way.

In college I filled out one of those forms and sent it off. I was already dating the man who is now my husband of more than twenty years. I thought it would be interesting to see who turned up and to find out what I was looking for. I also had this secret fantasy: What if he had done the same thing and we got picked as a match?

No such luck. In fact, I got back several letters from guys who sounded frighteningly like me. Their humor was identical to mine, only more exaggerated, it seemed to me. I prayed I would never meet them. I had no interest in someone who mirrored me, had reached all the same conclusions at such a young age, and had all my same faults!

You may remember Melissa from the Introduction, the girl who was constantly attracting cads who came on strong and romantic at first but were completely unreliable emotionally in a long-term relationship. She was a sanguine, always seeing the best in people and eager to relate. She was attracted to melancholics who often seemed like they needed someone strong and cheerful to help them achieve their passionate dreams of self-expression and freedom. Once she discovered it was the inspiration and intensity of these men, and not their neediness that was the real attraction, she was able to be more selective in the relationships she pursued. In other words, she looked for melancholics who had some balance and health rather than those who would immediately become dependent on her steady energy and positive thinking.

You may find it interesting to consider how so many of our games are based on four players. Eventually, each takes on one of the four temperaments. There's the leader, the responsible detail person, the communicative cheerleader person, and the melodramatic person. Even if these are not their temperaments in life in general, they will take on the roles if the game lasts long enough. Does it last because they fall into complementary humoral roles, or do they fall into the roles because the game must go on? (It has been said that time and causation are simply human inventions to help us make sense of the incomprehensible—is my sanguine showing?)

If the humoral roles adopted do not suit the players, if they are not at least their subdominant humors, the group will probably not gather again or at least not become a regular group. Sometimes, though, as one of the great attractions of games, you can play with a recessive humor in the context of a game and not have any serious consequences or have to change your whole character for good. For example, a phlegmatic person may enjoy playing the melodramatic melancholic person for an hour or two. Or she may take on the domineering choleric role, perhaps as the aggressive landlord in a Monopoly game.

How often in a game have you heard, "Hey, I've never seen that side of you before!" Or perhaps, "Wow, I've never seen you like this!"

Quartets that prove to be lasting almost always do so with four people who are complementary in their temperaments. It's fun to examine foursomes in our culture and figure out which represents which humor. If you watch the movie *Titanic*, for example, watch the four members of the quartet that plays music as the ship sinks. See if you can identify their dominant humors as they start to break up and then decide to keep on playing. It can be fascinating.

Take a look at just a few of the most famous people here and then think of others on your own. You may never look at rock groups, bridge tables, or movies with leading man/leading lady/supporting man/supporting lady the same way ever again.

Take the Beatles. John was the choleric, the solid, quiet, leader type. He had the vision, ultimately, to produce world peace. Paul was his phlegmatic counterpart. Cute as could be, a little on the soft side, never grew old, focused on love and family. George was the melancholic, tall and lanky, lean of face, with an obvious dark and mystical side. I thought I was being a rebel by saying I liked George when we high school girls all asked each other the burning question of the day, "Who's your favorite Beatle?" Most people chose Paul or John because they were better looking. Later, when I learned to pay attention to the humors, it became sadly obvious that as a decided sanguine, I would naturally be attracted to a George type over Paul or John.

Ringo, on the other hand, held no romantic attraction for me. I loved his wit and gentle aloofness, but as if he were a brother, not a romantic prospect. He was the sanguine partner, not tall or lean, but playful, ready for fun, with a certain raw sexiness. He has had the most to say in later years about the human condition and the healing of relationships, like a typical person of the sanguine temperament.

How about Dorothy, the Tin Man, the Lion, and the Scarecrow on their way to the Land of Oz? Can you guess?

The Lion is fairly obvious, the king of the jungle, wanting to get his courage to be the choleric leader he was meant to be.

The Tin Man is the melancholic fellow, made of metal, like minerals from the earth, wanting to get in touch with his heart, his creative, passionate inner being, to liberate himself from his cool, dry exterior and his fear of water and rust.

Scarecrow is the sanguine, wanting to find his brain, stuck in being silly, making people laugh with his goofiness and caring, but longing to explore the higher things in life with the sanguine proclivity for deep mental activity and brilliant communication.

Dorothy was the phlegmatic, the most childlike, inquisitive, and rebellious, but also doggedly dedicated to home and family and fairness, steadfast in her resolve, eager to help people, attentive to detail and the needs of others, outraged by betrayal, looking for security and home.

What about when Harry met Sally in the film of that name? Harry was the sanguine, preoccupied with sex, with early receding hair. Sally was the melancholic beauty, insecure but opinionated, changeable as the weather. Their friends who double-dated with them, and discovered each other when they had no attraction for Harry or Sally, are representative of the choleric man and the phlegmatic woman. Remember how angry Jess became over the wheel coffee table? He wanted his way in pure choleric fashion.

Remember how hung up his future wife was on one man who obviously wasn't going to leave his wife for her? Sound like perhaps an overly loyal phlegmatic who is not excited about change?

Take any foursome that works and chances are you will quickly discover that if their interactions ring true and are lasting, the four humors have created a lock among them.

I have a foursome of friends who have met together regularly for more than twelve years. Even when others join us we feel there is a special bond between us four. We are from different geographic and professional backgrounds, are at different ages and stages of life. When we first met, two of us were training for a modeling competition in New York (me a sanguine and Natalie a melancholic), and two of us were the trainers (Carol a choleric and Pat a phlegmatic). A common interest in modeling at the ripe age of twenty-five or over was about all we had in common. I suspect being the four oldest people in the room drew us together initially. But we've stuck together through thick and thin, literally as well as figuratively, and have taken great pleasure in each other, through births, deaths, marriage, divorce, careers and no careers, and more. We are classic representatives of the four humors. As different as four characters could get. And we love it. It is always interesting to get together.

The best actresses and actors can transform themselves from one type to another for the sake of a role. It is often uncanny. Take Laurence Olivier, for example. In *Henry V* he was born to be king, a young choleric who developed into his calling on the battle field. In *Hamlet,* he was a pining, self-absorbed melancholic. In *Richard III,* he was a scheming, sexually smarmy sanguine. In *Love Among the Ruins* with Katharine Hepburn as a spurned, domineering former lover, it is arguable that he played a phlegmatic, meticulous, masterful lawyer, against her vengeful choleric character. Hepburn too has played all roles with astounding skill and understanding.

Here are some famous romantic character pairs in film to further familiarize yourself with humoral matches. Consider Sally Fields and Paul Newman in *Verdict,* as phlegmatic and choleric characters. Leonardo DiCaprio and Kate Winslet in *Titanic* were melancholic and sanguine, the artist and the adventurer. In *Gone With the Wind,* Clark Gable was the sanguine and Vivien Leigh the melancholic, the sexy adventurer, and the beautiful but inconsistent devourer of life.

How about Jack Lemmon and Marilyn Monroe in *Some Like It Hot*? Again sanguine and melancholic. Lucille Ball and Desi Arnez in *I Love Lucy* were choleric wife, tall, controlling, wanting to be number one, desirous to be the lead on the stage, and phlegmatic husband, smaller, lovable, highly skilled, loyal, eager to please, consistent, always playing tricks to get back at her for her ambition. His Cuban temper and her melodramatic weeping were all the more "humorous" because they were out of character with the basic relationship, as were their circumstances. There was absolutely endless fertile ground for problems because of these mismatches. Fred and Ethel played the sanguine and melancholic neighbors, him always with the roving eye complaining about Ethel's lack of interest in sex and Ethel always coming up with plots and problems for Lucille, her leader, to solve.

These actors are not necessarily typecast. They may not be in real life, in their physical attributes or their personalities, good representatives of the humoral temperaments they portray. Instead, their personalities in these particular relationships exhibited these humors. Great actors knowingly or unknowingly key into their complementary humors or their keen observation of others to show romantic "chemistry" on stage.

Other groups to have fun with are The Honeymooners; Mickey, Minnie, Donald, and Goofy; the four Marx Brothers; and so on.

On a much more serious note, consider the four versions of Jesus in the four Gospels of the Bible. In Matthew, Jesus has a commanding authority that others obey (choleric). In Mark, Jesus is a passionate but unappreciated helper to the people (melancholic). In Luke, Jesus is teacher and healer (sanguine). In John, he is the Son sent on a mission of sacrifice (phlegmatic). It has been remarked that only with four Gospels could we get the full picture of Jesus' magnificence. It may be enlightening to consider that one reason Jesus remains so hard to pin down is because he offers a perfect balance, with appeal to all temperamental types.

If you discover your best friend does not match you in the classic complementary pairs, don't worry. Awareness is 90 percent of the challenge. Perfect complementarity is virtually impossible anyhow because of the subordinate humoral patterns and relative proportions of the influences of each. Other factors play a part too. But if you can recognize quickly your differences as well as your common values and concerns, you can avoid a huge number of small insults and larger conflicts between you.

Take the case of the choleric businessperson, for example, who wishes his sanguine business partner were more compliant rather than argumentative. When he remembers their shared interest in control and in ideas, they can aim to accomplish something together as partners rather than seek to control each other.

It is interesting to note that once you choose a complementary humor as a best friend, you may be drawn to a different-type humoral temperament for other relationships.

For example, for mentors or personal coaches you might do best with those who share your own dominant humor, assuming they are in relatively healthy balance. You may not be physically or even emotionally attracted to them, but you may discover that they have an uncanny understanding of your life challenges, habitual emotional responses, values, and ways of expressing yourself. They may be able to get through to you when others can't. This can be extremely valuable, and time- and cost-serving as well.

Figures 10 through 16 will give you some more ideas about how the humors play out in relationships.

With a growing understanding of how your temperament affects your relationships, your romantic life and friendships can take a quantum leap.

♠ C	S ♥
Control Body Action Group dynamics Power Winning Competition Best Results Accomplishment	Cooperation Spirit Interaction Communication Intention Control Society Process Progress Relationships
Competition Mind Efficiency Thought Art Systems Variety Creativity Freedom Facts	Responsibility Heart Security Freedom Loyalty Consistency Cooperation Fun Family Attitude
♦ M	P ♣

FIGURE 10. **Key Concerns.** These are topics these people will enjoy talking about most and will look for in the people they enjoy being around. Notice that the choleric and melancholic share competitiveness. The sanguine and choleric share interest in control and authority. The sanguine and phlegmatic share a liking for cooperative endeavor. The melancholic and phlegmatic share an interest in freedom. This shows how different alliances can form in any group and common concerns can bind any pair to common efforts and goals. The trick is to recognize these commonalities so that they can be used as a foundation for mutually beneficial relationships.

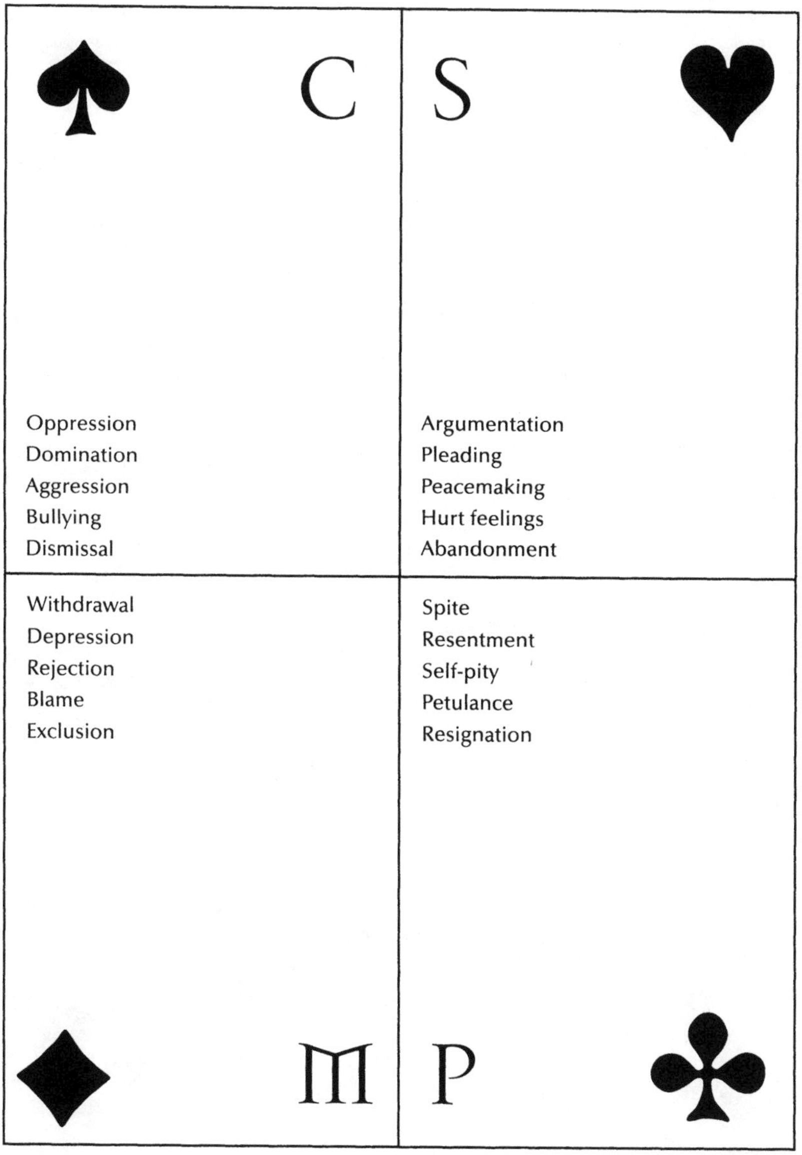

♠ C	S ♥
Oppression	Argumentation
Domination	Pleading
Aggression	Peacemaking
Bullying	Hurt feelings
Dismissal	Abandonment
Withdrawal	Spite
Depression	Resentment
Rejection	Self-pity
Blame	Petulance
Exclusion	Resignation
◆ M	P ♣

FIGURE 11. Dominant Reaction to Conflict in a Relationship.
Unfortunately conflict can bring out the worst in people if they are out of balance. If you experience one of these clusters in someone you care about, consider beginning your response by addressing one of their concerns listed in Figure 10 that is relevant to the troublesome situation. Meanwhile, try to avoid reacting from your own cluster of temperamental responses. Habits die hard, but if you develop a better alternative, they are easier to shake off.

♠ C	S ♥
Grand surprises Pride Quick action Declaration Future projection Grand vision	Compliments Parties Fast talk Passion Building bonds Connection
Jubilance Playfulness Spontaneity Gifts Grand plans Music	Gratitude Smiles Appreciation Fantasy Games Laughter
♦ M	P ♣

FIGURE 12. **Ways of Showing Joy in Relationships.** These clusters help show you the temperament of the person you are with. They can also help you to share in their joy when you otherwise would not fully appreciate it, expecting them to express joy the way you do. Likewise, you can better share your joy if you allow room in your day for their own way of sharing your joy. For example, a phlegmatic may want to focus on giving credit where it's due after a great accomplishment, while the melancholic may want to make jokes at the hero's expense. There can be room for both.

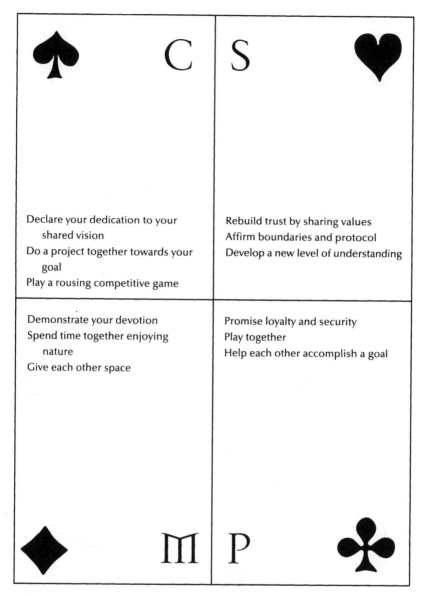

♠ C	S ♥
Declare your dedication to your shared vision Do a project together towards your goal Play a rousing competitive game	Rebuild trust by sharing values Affirm boundaries and protocol Develop a new level of understanding
Demonstrate your devotion Spend time together enjoying nature Give each other space	Promise loyalty and security Play together Help each other accomplish a goal
♦ ♏	P ♣

FIGURE 13. **Preferred Way of Making Up—Reconciliation.** These differences can be crucial in a relationship. A conflict will not feel like it's over until both parties have accomplished their humoral style of reconciliation. Insisting on your way first may be counterproductive. Rather, ask for a multiple-solution approach that will make you both feel better and help you get back in good humor.

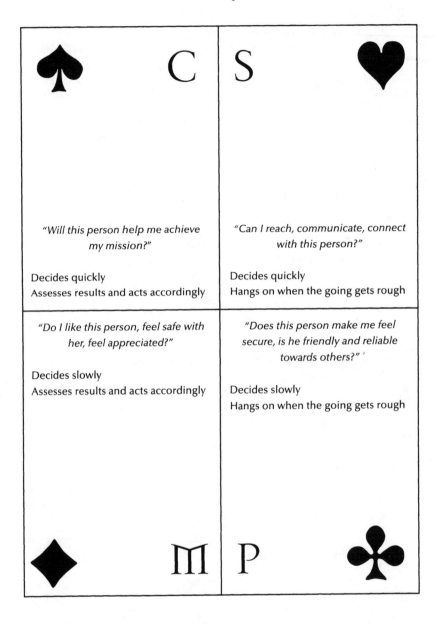

FIGURE 14. **Decision-Making about Relationships.** Most of us have conversations with ourselves or a close confidant about our relationships. What questions do we ask ourselves? What answers do we look for? Each temperament has a different question. Who might give the desired answer, based on your knowledge of the humors so far?

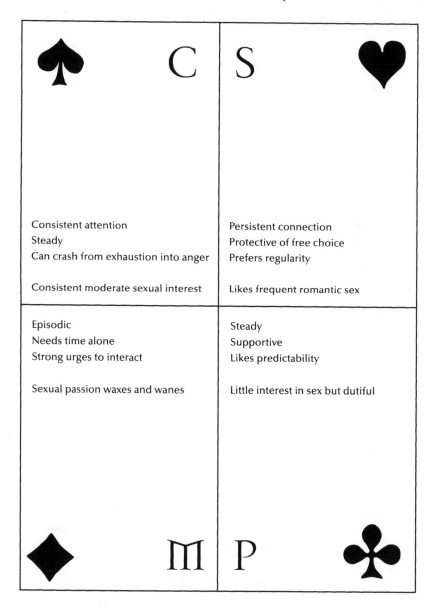

♠ C | S ♥

Consistent attention
Steady
Can crash from exhaustion into anger

Consistent moderate sexual interest

Persistent connection
Protective of free choice
Prefers regularity

Likes frequent romantic sex

Episodic
Needs time alone
Strong urges to interact

Sexual passion waxes and wanes

Steady
Supportive
Likes predictability

Little interest in sex but dutiful

♦ Ⅲ | P ♣

Figure 15. Rhythms of Relationships. Each temperament has its own habitual rhythm. It can be particularly useful to recognize these in your friends and loved ones. Being clear about your own rhythms can also help prevent misunderstandings and unintended slights to your partner or associate. Consider in particular the differences in rhythms of sexual appetite. When the natural flexibility associated with humoral balance is lacking, these differences can destroy a relationship.

C S	
♠	♥
I see ... You can see that ... I want ... desire—action	I understand ... It feels like ... I sense ... feeling—communications
I hear you ... Listen to me ... I know ... knowledge—information	I'm touched that... I wish ... I believe ... belief—experience
♦	♣
ℼ P	

FIGURE 16. **Favorite Words and Phrases.** How we say things is as important as what we say in getting our point across to another person. It may be more important as far as creating a bond that can be a foundation for future interactions, because how we say it expresses something profound about our being, our humoral spirit. Raise your antennas in your next conversation so you can notice not just what people say but how they say it. Notice how you may already be drawing conclusions unconsciously about "where they are coming from." Now you can become more conscious about these cues and therefore perhaps more effective and congenial in your chosen response.

[In Shakespeare's *Henry IV* plays] Falstaff, Pistol, Bardolph, and the rest of the gang were themselves "humor" characters, and in the list of persons printed in the first folio in 1623 are labeled "irregular humorists." . . .

Jonson was a student of the classics. He approved Aristotle's theories of drama . . . . Moreover, he held, as did most serious critics of the time, that all literature had a moral purpose. The particular purpose of comedy was to chastise folly by making it ridiculous. Accordingly, in his plays he created characters which were contemporary types, and so plotted the story that each "humor" displays his own particular folly and is suitably punished for it. . . .

Every Man <u>out</u> of His Humor was a failure. After the success of *Every Man <u>in</u> His Humor,* Jonson became very arrogant, and he prefaced the new play with an induction or introductory piece in which three characters, apparently spectators, come onto the stage to discuss his theory of the humors and the purpose and history of comedy. The play itself was not so good as its predecessor; the portraits of the humors were too exact and the plot too involved.

—HARRISON, G. B., "General Introduction,"
in Harrison, *Shakespeare (1564–1616),*
The Complete Works, pp. 41–43 (underlines added)

CHAPTER 6

Your Humoral Calling:
Career Choices by the Humors

Only the man who is still animal is governed, mastered, compelled, driven by the stars, so that he has no choice but to follow them—just as the thief cannot escape the gallows . . . the game the hunter. But the reason for all this is that such a man does not know himself and does not know how to use the energies hidden in him, nor does he know that he carries the stars within himself, that he is the microcosm, and thus carries in him the whole firmament with all its influences. . . .

The wisdom of Christ is more profound than that of nature, consequently a prophet or an apostle must be held in higher esteem than an astronomer or a physician, and it is better to prophesy from God than through astronomy, it is better to cure through God than by means of herbs. . . . Nevertheless it is our duty to say that the sick need a physician, while few need an apostle; similarly many forecasts must be made by the astronomer and not by the prophets. Thus each has his part—the prophet, the astronomer, the apostle, and the physician. For this reason astronomy has not been abolished, nor forbidden to us Christians; we have only been commanded to use it in a Christian manner. For the Father has set us in the light of nature, and the Son in the eternal light. Therefore it is indispensable that we should know them both.

—PARACELSUS, "German Practice from the Year 1538," and "About Knowledge of the Stars," in Jacobi, *Paracelsus: Selected Writings*, pp. 1537–41

MAGINE YOUR OWN work environment, and think of it as a team of people with a common goal to accomplish. It will be very helpful to have all humors represented, even though you will not get along with some as easily as with others. We are taught to admire leaders and to all learn to be "leaders," but in any situation of group effort, not everyone should be a leader. A phlegmatic person may be very comfortable and happy as a fine leader in his family, but in his work situation he may be the absolutely essential anchor and detail person for his organization. An effective, happy choleric person may learn to be a cooperative, supportive person with his choleric son or his melancholic daughter. Or perhaps at a restaurant, he may be ready to indulge his phlegmatic receptive, fun side, rather than keeping control and leadership and telling the server exactly what to do, embarrassing his tablemates.

In fact all humoral temperaments will show superior status or leadership at some time or another, but with a subtle but profound difference in focus, a difference in what you might call leadership style or purpose. Figure 17 illustrates these different styles of leadership. The choleric is the most comfortable as a commander. In situations that require quick decisions, huge vision, and decisive action, a commander may be essential.

The phlegmatic leads as a master. The master draws apprentices to him and shares his craft and artistry by doing, by example, demonstrating his mastery through discipline, persistence, and concentration. Masters do their craft and attract their followers to them because of their ability to produce results.

The sanguine leads as a wizard. The wizard takes people on a journey, an adventure. She creates situations in which the willing

♠ C	S ♥
Commander Leads by vision Offers clarity Attracts by dominance	Wizard Leads by sharing an adventure Offers good sense Attracts by enthusiasm
Sage Leads by superior knowledge Offers analysis Attracts by inspiration	Master Leads by example Offers pragmatism Attracts by team
♦ M	P ♣

FIGURE 17. **Styles of Leadership.** The choleric is the classic leader, but each temperament can lead in his or her own way. And each must be a follower as well as a leader to be educated in the path to pursue. Note that the commander declares a goal and enrolls people in the vision. The wizard creates magic and offers a well-guided tour of mystery. The sage waits on the hillside for the student to appear. The master surrounds his or her work with a group who admire the skill and persistence exhibited. The sage and master wait for their following, while the commander and wizard actively seek them out.

student learns. The sanguine's followers are attracted by the spirit and mystery of the wizard. She amazes and at the same time empowers her students.

The melancholic leads as a sage. Her wisdom attracts the multitudes. Her mercurial temperament is overlooked by her followers in order to absorb the knowledge and information the sage has gathered through rich and varied experience. Followers come and go as they reach their desired level of enlightenment.

The wizard moves your spirit to intention, the sage moves your mind to understanding and a plan, the master moves the heart to commitment to skills and discipline, and the commander moves the body to action. What organization would not benefit from having these four kinds of leaders on tap?

The most successful people in fact are very flexible. They are both aware of their own appropriate role in any situation and of the tendencies of those around them, so that they can accomplish their common goals and get along well together in the process.

How might this information help you in dealing with a coworker, neighbor, or supervisor?

Career choices begin in schooling. Your school performance can actually be thought of as your first career. Even if you think you know what you want to be when you grow up, sometimes your performance at school affects how quickly or how effectively you get where you want to go. Consider for a moment, what your temperament can tell you about your school experience. If the learning style offered in your school experience was a mismatch with your temperament, it may be liberating to realize that future career opportunities that are in harmony with your temperament need not be limited by your past educational experiences; your achievement level may be very different from your school performance. This is often noted in studies of how school predicts career success. If you pick a career function that suits your humors, you will excel.

Figure 18 shows the various learning styles characteristic of the four humoral temperaments.

As you move as a young adult into the marketplace, consider what it could mean to be more aware of the humors. If you were

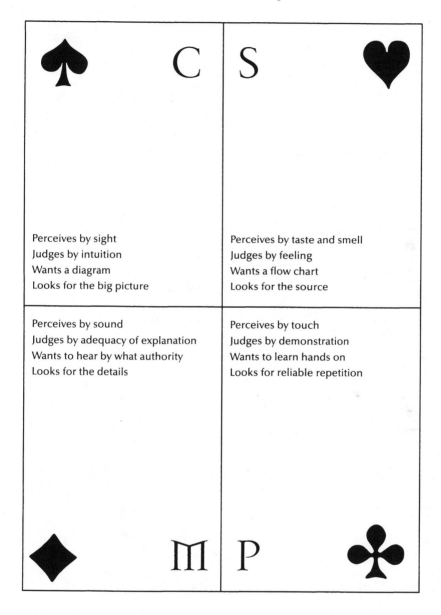

Perceives by sight
Judges by intuition
Wants a diagram
Looks for the big picture

Perceives by taste and smell
Judges by feeling
Wants a flow chart
Looks for the source

Perceives by sound
Judges by adequacy of explanation
Wants to hear by what authority
Looks for the details

Perceives by touch
Judges by demonstration
Wants to learn hands on
Looks for reliable repetition

FIGURE 18. **Favorite Style of Learning and Information Processing.**
Jungian theory has highlighted different methods of learning as a distinguishing
characteristic of the four basic types. These observations go back thousands of years
in the association of the humors with the various senses and tastes.

The Vocabulary
of Humorology
in Everyday Life

In **THE APPENDIX** to his anthology *Shakespeare, The Complete Works,* G. B. Harrison summarizes the impact of the humors on the English language and culture this way:

> Anatomy was much studied toward the end of the sixteenth century, and the word became popular in literary jargon to denote what is now called analysis or psychology. When learned men examined the human body, they were impressed by its all-pervading humor or quality of dampness. But the "humors" of the body were obviously of different kinds, and on the assumption the physical body must be composed of four elements, "earth" was identified as black bile, etc. . . . Each element produced a corresponding temperament. . . .
>
> In the 1590s the word "humor" rapidly became popular, as words sometimes will, and every intelligent person began to talk of his humors. Indeed, it became the mark of a would-be intellectual to have a humor, preferably melancholic, which was the sign of a great mind. . . .
>
> In Shakespeare's plays the word "humor" is very common and has a wide range of meanings. It may be used literally to mean moisture, or to imply one of the four humors, but its commonest meanings are whim, obsession, temperament, mood, temper, or inclination. (pp. 1632–33).

Here is a selection of words and phrases that are part of our cultural heritage from the humors and temperaments. They illustrate how the humors permeate our culture, mostly without our knowing it. The echoes of trained intuition, down through the ages, are there to enrich our understanding.

Humor—That quality of being funny, comical. Derived from farce and comedy based on exaggerated portrayals of the humors of various dramatic characters in the dramatic productions of Elizabethan England, around 1600.

In good humor—Feeling good. Derived from being in a good balance with your humors, the four natural ethereal forces of life, associated with the basic elements of the universe.

Humorous—Being funny or amusing. Derived from being a reflection of your humors and therefore amusing to those around you. See "humor" above.

In bad humor—Difficult to be with. Derived from being out of balance, showing the bad side of your dominant humor.

The good humor man—Someone who gives you something that puts you in a good humor. Ice cream has cream for the sanguines, sugar for the melancholics, and milk for the phlegmatics. Cholerics usually go for the hamburger or hot dog.

Ill-humored—Being out of balance, bad attitude, humors out of sorts. (Is there a connection here? We "sort" playing cards, and we are in bad humor when we are "out of sorts." How far can we go with this?)

Bad-tempered—Also "ill-tempered." In a bad mood, difficult to get along with. Easily angered or provoked. Not congenial or a good sport. Out of our proper temperament.

Suit, as in "That suits you," "Suit yourself," "It doesn't suit me"—Something that appears to fit or match well with your personality or style. Derived from the French for follow or flow, "suivre." The same word used for the four designations for a deck of cards. These suits have corresponded to the humors since ancient times. Does your suit suit you? That is, does it flatter your humoral gifts?

Influence—The power to make something change without physical force. Derived from the fluids or humors, which were thought in ancient times to influence all matter and life.

Bilious—Complaining, aggressively angry. Derived from the bile presumed to bring on the domineering mood of the choleric humor.

Hot-blooded—Passionate. Showing an excess of the sanguine humor.

Flu—An invisible, invasive disease. Derived from "influenza," old terminology about the danger of bad humors or fluids overcoming the healthy body in inclement environments.

Cold—Why is a cold called a cold? We know it's not the night air or the cold, that cause our distress, but airborne or hand-borne viruses and molds to which our bodies react immuno-logically. But mothers today can still be heard to say, "Look out, you'll catch your death of cold." The ancient meaning would be, "Cold is going to be the death of you," as opposed to heat, wetness, or dryness.

Sanguine—Still used to mean someone with a cheerful, some-times Pollyanna disposition.

Melancholic—Still used to mean someone feeling depressed and sad.

Choleric—Rarely heard but still used occasionally to refer to a hot temper. It is interesting that even though "cholesterol" is made by the liver every day and is essential for hormones, immune factors, and skin integrity, it has been made into the bad guy with very little evidence, at least partly by relying on this cultural distrust of anything having to do with "choler." But now we know there is good cholesterol and bad choles-terol, just as there are balanced as well as imbalanced cholerics. If you are in a disaster area, pray that a balanced choleric is running things.

Phlegmatic—Still used to mean lethargic, slow to react.

Humor me!—Meaning play up to me just as I am, indulge me in my wants and preferences. A direct reference to the ancient humors. Even gets said on occasional TV sitcoms.

Influential—Someone who is influential is able to exert power without force by appealing to the nature of the person being influenced—in other words, by working with, instead of against, the unseen "flow" of the universal forces.

Influenza—The flu. We know it is not from bad air or nasty vapors but rather viruses spread by a handshake or a sneeze or unclean food. Yet the term still harkens back over a hundred years to the idea of a malignant vapor imbalancing our health.

Humoral—In medicine the term is still used to describe the various influences at work at the cellular level, having to do with the constitution of the cellular tissue and the flow of biological substances. Here used to refer to the ancient wisdom of the humors.

Livery—A term still used in Britain to describe someone who has melancholic symptoms.

Fiery—When used to describe a fiery tongue or a fiery disposition, it is an inadvertent reference to the basic element of the choleric.

A sanguine complexion—Still means a bit ruddy, red from high circulation to the face. A bit flushed. Similar use with melancholic, meaning having a dark, moody visage.

Temperament—The personality or disposition of a person. The four humors were also called the four temperaments in Renaissance England, as in "he was of a phlegmatic temperament."

Constitution—The combination of the four humors forms the constitution of a person. How they are arranged, their ebb and flow, and their proportionality, combine to give you your constitution. You could have a strong constitution or a weak constitution depending on your susceptibility to disease or imbalance. A term used in homeopathy.

Disposition—Disposed to a certain temperament.

Vapors— As in, "Catch the vapors." Mysterious forces that can cause ill health. Another word for the humors.

Temper—Something you lose when you act out of anger or no longer have self-control. You "keep your temper" when you maintain self-control. Someone can "show his temper" when he gets angry, "choleric," or "bilious." Some still say "Don't show your temper!" to mean keep your overwrought humor to yourself. The temper actually refers to the delicate balance of your humors. Medieval physician Paracelsus called the four humors "tempers."

Putting on airs—Pretending that you are affected by some humor, especially melancholia, which has a certain chic to it, or did in Elizabethan England, around 1600.

Humorology—A new word. The study of the four humors, their history, their ancient masters, their literature, their connections to other systems of thought, and their impact on health, character, career, personality, relationships, lifestyle preferences, spirituality, balance, romance, and happiness.

Consider also: "Warm-hearted," "Cold-blooded," "Dry wit," "Cool-handed," "Wet and wild," and more. Perhaps all such expressions are not direct humoral references, but many of them are, and all of them conjure up deep humoral connections rooted in our collective consciousness about the very nature of our beings. Now that you have a familiarity with the humors, you may have a special appreciation for the wealth of wisdom and yes, humor, that lies within the humors and the language and imagery they have created.

being interviewed by a tall, sturdy-looking man with intent eyes and wide forehead and square chin, you would want to say something like, "I think I have the drive and vision to execute your purpose." You would do best not to say, "I'm good at being open with my feelings so that I can build trust and a cooperative environment." His choleric interest in achievement is much more important that a feeling of cooperation.

But the second statement might work well for a smaller, robust, talkative sort of interviewer who is phlegmatic.

If you are seeking cooperation from a tall, slender businesswoman, seeking some service, you would have more luck saying, "I know you are busy, but I would really appreciate it if you could you help me for a moment, as soon as you are ready." This would be much better than, "I wish you would help me because my train is leaving very soon." But that would do fine for a phlegmatic sort of store clerk. She would appreciate your predicament and move to help you. The melancholic is more motivated by your respect for her time and freedom of choice whether to help you, while the phlegmatic is inspired to help by your frank statement of need.

Granted it seems subtle, but your own wealth of experience already influences you to the better responses if you take some time to consider, even for a moment, who it is you are talking to and who you are seeking to move to action on your behalf. It will be as if you were training your natural intuition. Even a born pitcher needs coaching and practice.

What if you are not satisfied with the work you are doing? Can the humors help?

As you might imagine from the communications styles characteristic of the different temperaments and the variations in their chief concerns and preoccupations, people of different humors will be most content and stimulated by some careers more than others. The good news is that in today's marketplace, almost any arena of work or career offers a variety of functions or roles, so that you may not have to completely retrain for a different field even if you discover your dissatisfaction comes from being in the wrong kind of work.

For example, Michelle, who was mentioned in the Introduction, was very unhappy with her computer job. We identified her as characterized by the sanguine temperament. She wanted to be with people and feared she had chosen the wrong field. She had not really chosen it, she said. Rather it chose her because she was good in math and interested in computers as a communications medium and went along with her teachers in order to please them. Her sanguine tendencies led her to where she was, but the work did not nurture her better sanguine nature. I suggested she see what people-oriented functions were available in her company. Within a month she was doing training, teaching, and coaching about computers, and was in sanguine heaven, so to speak.

Another woman, a young mother named Joan, was a teacher, but felt she had burned out early. She loved children, but just didn't like the lesson plans, school administrative duties, and trying to maintain discipline with difficult kids. We discovered she was of the melancholic temperament. I asked her if she had ever thought about being an artist. She said she had always wanted to be one but was no good at it. I wondered how she knew that. She said her fifth grade teacher had told her so—absolutely no potential. "As a teacher now yourself, do you think that teacher should have said that?" Joan had an aha. "No . . . of course not. I would never want to limit a student like that." She started taking adult night school classes once a week in painting and this teacher said she had a gift! She became more mellow with her children and felt more at ease about her teaching. She felt she became a better teacher too and enjoyed it more.

Remember Sam and Mike, business partners from the Introduction? They had a law practice together. Sam was a melancholic and Mike was a sanguine. Sam got impatient easily and wanted the bottom-line result and Mike wanted to get the whole story and see how everything fit together with their long-term plans before making a decision. By accepting each other's humoral preferences, they found ways to shorten meetings for Sam's sake, to develop a mission statement and regular mileposts for Mike's sake, and to divide up information necessary for a decision in ways that each would enjoy the part of the analysis they were responsible for. Mutual respect grew as each could delegate to the other what they didn't enjoy doing and appreciate that the other did a good job on his part.

As a last example, let's take Sarah, the saleswoman who was constantly second-guessing her approach to people when a sale fell through. She was so eager for the sale that she tried many different techniques, but she failed to find out what humoral personality she was dealing with in each case, so the technique seldom matched the prospect. A classic portrayal of this situation is the efforts of the Ann Benning character in the film *American Beauty*, when she set out to make a sale at her real estate open house event. Each strategy fell on deaf ears because it didn't match the prospect. In Sarah's case, when Sarah realized she was a choleric and tended toward aggressive and forceful behavior, she realized that few buyers would respond well to this style, no matter what the verbal strategy. She also learned to start slowly with each new customer, so that she could intuit their particular humoral character. Then she could go slow with phlegmatics and sanguines, give the bottom line with melancholics, talk about family with the phlegmatics and fun with the sanguines and vision with the melancholics. When she had a choleric, she knew exactly what to do. They matched up quickly and she could make a quick deal.

Figure 19 gives career tendencies for each humor, including classic and contemporary possibilities. But again, most important is what regular functions you do in your chosen field to get daily satisfaction. If you want a complete change of careers, surely go for it. But be careful not to slip into a function within that field that still does not meet your temperament. Figures 20 and 21 depict some humoral types in rewarding professions suitable to their temperaments.

Now that you have had an opportunity in the last couple of chapters to absorb useful information about how the humors affect your relationships at home, among friends, and at work, we can move on to personal and lifestyle preferences that manifest the humoral balances.

<table>
<tr><td>

♠   C</td><td>S   ♥</td></tr>
</table>

♠ C	S ♥
Military general Sports team captain Statesman Politician CEO **Building**	Military strategist Team defender Teacher Minister Orator **Communication**
Military analyst Team hero Artist Performer Scientist **Rules and breaking the rules**	Military regular Team anchor Craftsperson Counselor Social worker **Causes and communities**
◆ Ⅲ	P ♣

FIGURE 19. **Favorite Careers.** Associating temperaments with different careers goes back several millennia. The exercise has been used to limit people's options as often as to encourage them to follow their dreams. In almost any field of endeavor in which you find yourself, there are aspects that can be emphasized to bring about greater satisfaction by humoring your innate talents and gifts. If you feel a need to expand your horizons, consider a field where your temperamental proclivities are front and center. All can be entrepreneurs in the new economy, but to be successful and happy at it, each must attract people to help them who are complementary in their innate skill sets so each can do what they like to do best in their chosen field.

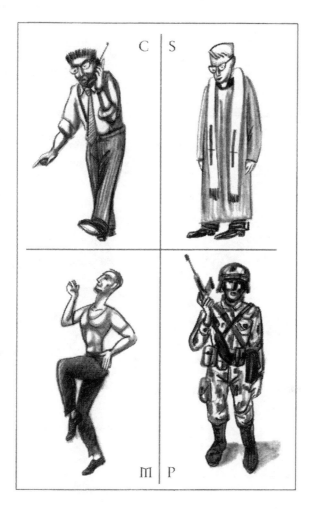

FIGURE 20. Favorite Careers by the Humors—Four Men. These men have chosen careers likely to agree with their natural inclinations according to temperament. Cholerics like to manage. Phlegmatics like to help. Sanguines like to teach. Melancholics like to perform. Illustrations by Robert Rayevsky.

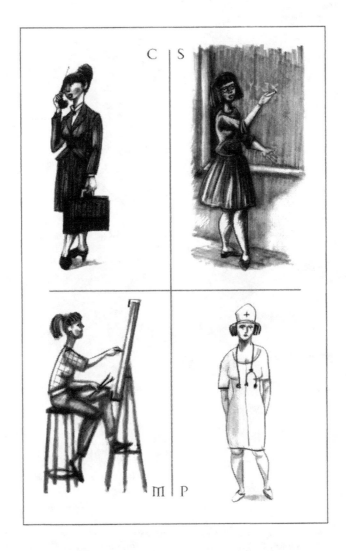

FIGURE 21. Favorite Careers by the Humors—Four Women. You can see how much fun it can be to use the humors in developing characters for plays and stories. What we sometimes call stereotypes can be damaging when they limit people from making their own choices or judge one career to be less presitgious or important than another. But many stereotypes can ring true to our intuition because according to the concept of the humors, some are more temperamentally suited to some kinds of occupation than are others, not as a limitation but as a way to maximize their own satisfaction. The key is to keep in mind that no outside authority should decide but only the job seekers themselves. Illustrations by Robert Rayevsky.

The ancients themselves, Chaucer, and other later writers had made free use of psychology in their determination of motive and in their description of the passions of the mind. In the last quarter of the sixteenth century there arose a far wider realization of the possibilities of psychology and a far greater faith in what it might accomplish. Timothy Bright and Robert Burton applied it to the diagnosis and cure of insanity. John Huarte offered it as a method by which men might be classified for trades and professions, through a determination of the proportions in them of the qualities of hot, cold, moist, and dry. Besides these there was a great group of writers, partly scientific and partly popular, who saw in psychological phenomena, often called "humours," a means of explaining and depicting the emotional life of man. The subject passed from the scientist to the literary man, just as we have seen pragmatism and psychoanalysis pass in our own day. Shakespeare and nearly all the dramatists became psychologists, and according to their ability and genius, made use of psychology in their plays.

—HARDIN CRAIG, "General Introduction," in Craig,
The Complete Works of Shakespeare (1564–1616), p. 12

Your Humoral Behaviors:
Food, Energy, and Lifestyle by the Humors

The body has four kinds of taste—the sour, the sweet, the bitter, and the salty. . . . They are to be found in every creature, but only in man can they be studied. . . . Everything bitter is hot and dry, that is to say, choleric; everything sour is cold and dry, that is to say, melancholic. . . . The sweet gives rise to the phlegmatic, for everything sweet is cold and moist, even though it must not be compared to water. . . . The sanguine originates in the salty, which is hot and moist. . . . If the salty predominates in man as compared with the three others, he is sanguine; if the bitter is predominant in him, he is choleric. The sour makes him melancholic, and the sweet, if it predominates, phlegmatic. Thus the four tempers are rooted in the body of man as in garden mould.

—PARACELSUS (1493–1541), "The Birth of Man," and "The Qualities of Man,"
in Jacobi, *Paracelsus: Selected Writings*, pp. 19–20

I N READING THIS book so far, you have heard mostly about constitutional tendencies in physique and character created by whichever humor dominates in the personal makeup of each person. Now as you read on, you can gain a deeper understanding of how your personal preferences and lifestyle choices profoundly affect the way the humors manifest in thought, behavior, and emotions.

The best thing about these lifestyle tastes and preferences is that unlike physical characteristics, habitual emotional tendencies, and deep attractive forces in relationships, which you cannot change easily if at all, the qualities you will hear about in this and the next few chapters can be deliberately altered, adjusted, and evolved. And it is often easy, fun, effective, and sometimes dramatic to do so.

What is your favorite snack food?

It is no accident that pizza, ice cream, fried chicken, and potato chips are the most popular foods on the American market, or that beer and soda are the most popular drinks, although now apparently we must add coffees.

Because we have been ignorant of the importance of a dynamic balance of our humors, the internal forces of life, you and I and most of America have been propelled into a cycle of exaggerated humoral response and cravings for quick input and stimulation to rebalance or jump-start those forces.

Please note the accompanying chart, Figure 22. It's one of the most important in the book. It not only tells you a lot about yourself if you combine it with what has gone before, but it also gives you the key to solving innumerable problems big and small that

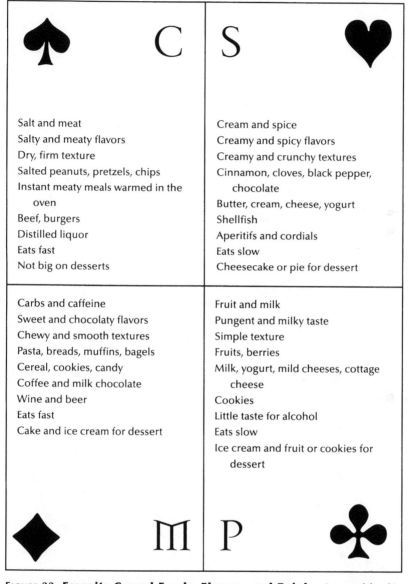

♠ C	S ♥
Salt and meat Salty and meaty flavors Dry, firm texture Salted peanuts, pretzels, chips Instant meaty meals warmed in the oven Beef, burgers Distilled liquor Eats fast Not big on desserts	Cream and spice Creamy and spicy flavors Creamy and crunchy textures Cinnamon, cloves, black pepper, chocolate Butter, cream, cheese, yogurt Shellfish Aperitifs and cordials Eats slow Cheesecake or pie for dessert
Carbs and caffeine Sweet and chocolaty flavors Chewy and smooth textures Pasta, breads, muffins, bagels Cereal, cookies, candy Coffee and milk chocolate Wine and beer Eats fast Cake and ice cream for dessert	Fruit and milk Pungent and milky taste Simple texture Fruits, berries Milk, yogurt, mild cheeses, cottage cheese Cookies Little taste for alcohol Eats slow Ice cream and fruit or cookies for dessert
♦ M	P ♣

FIGURE 22. **Favorite Craved Foods, Flavors, and Drinks.** A craved food is one you will eat more of when you know you have had enough, or one you will fantasize about when you are under stress or too busy to eat, even though you know a healthy mini-meal would help you more. These foods feed your dominant humor and therefore can throw you more off balance if you indulge in them when you cannot balance them with other foods or with appropriate changes in environmental conditions or physical activity. You may notice that all the empty calorie foods today aim at one or more humors and so find a persistent market among those ignorant of the value of maintaining their humoral balance.

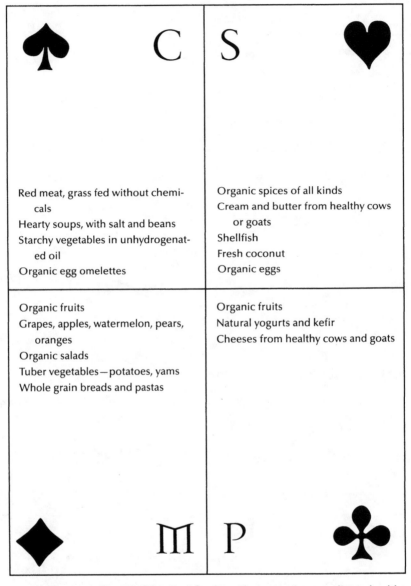

FIGURE 23. Favorite Healthy Foods. Even if you restrict your diet to healthy foods, you can still imbalance your humors by going after the wrong foods at the wrong times, though it is a lot harder than with the concentrated junk foods available today to feed your overwrought humors directly. The good news is that some simple corrections can allow for better balance without your giving up your favorite healthy foods. These include watching the time of day for your humors and taking balancing foods such as steamed or fresh organic vegetables and fruits and grains with a low glycemic index.

can occur in your life, as you shall come to see, hear, sense, and experience further along.

As you will see from Figure 23, even if you eat quite well, from all-natural, whole, home-prepared foods, there are still natural preferences associated with the humors, which if eaten in excess to the exclusion of other foods can cause imbalances that will show up in personality and mood as well as weight distribution and even, as you will hear later, disease patterns.

If you want to know why these basic dietary preferences can make such a difference, you can consider a variety of explanations, ranging from the ancient association with the four natural elements, fire, air, earth, and water, to the scientific association of the humors with the various hormone-producing glands you met before in the discussion of developmental physiology, or why we look the way we do.

Let's take a look at both approaches.

The Choleric Metabolism

FROM THE ANCIENT mystical point of view, the choleric humor is associated with the sun, with the qualities of heat and dryness. This humor then has affinity with foods that create heat and dryness in the body. Contraction is one way to generate heat and dryness. Red meats and sodium or salt have this effect. Red meats are the most concentrated package of protein and fat together with the vitamins and minerals that build up body heat. They cause the body to build concentrated tissue in the form of muscle. Salt also dries and concentrates the body by pulling water out of the tissues. People of the choleric temperament get thirsty very easily and sweat profusely.

From the scientific point of view, the choleric humor is associated with the adrenal glands. These glands produce hormones that help you respond to stress. Stress is defined as any condition inside or outside of the body that requires a shift from resting homeostasis or internal balance of the body. That is, any adjustment that is required for the well-being of the organism. The adrenal hormones speed heart rate, breathing, and muscular enervation, to allow the body to flee or fight for quick self-preservation. Today most stresses don't require fight or flight but must be handled in more subtle ways. Many experts assume this is why stress builds up in the body. But others believe that our bodies can handle all kinds of subtle stresses if the body is in balance energetically so that adjustments can be made without major distortion of key functions of the body.

To make the shifts possible, the adrenal glands also suppress rational mental function, digestion, pain sensation, and other internal functions that would divert energy and distract the organism—that's you—away from the necessary response to a crisis. The adrenal hormones activate the sympathetic nervous system, which contracts the muscles for action.

Salt and red meat are the most powerful foods for stimulating the adrenal glands. Distilled alcohol also seems to have this effect. Remember the cowboy movies, with shots of whiskey, macho men asserting their manhood, and endless brawling with no sign of normal pain response?

Meanwhile, the adrenal glands need extra vitamin C to maintain integrity under stress, as well as the B vitamins and trace minerals.

You may find it interesting to know that people dominant in the choleric humor are extremely resilient to stress, especially when young. They seem to be able to go non stop all day, often with very little sleep.

About four or five o'clock, their energy droops. Is it that the circadian or natural daily rhythm of the adrenals is to slow down in the afternoon, or is it that the sun, the power of the choleric humor, is beginning to go down at that time of day?

Does it matter which? Or are they actually related or identical forces? I will leave that to your own metaphysical imagination. Meanwhile, both fit fine.

That time in the afternoon is when the choleric dominant person often wants a hearty cocktail, like a martini, a salty vodka drink, or a steak for dinner, to get her or him through the evening. If she gets it, she can sustain a few more hours of activity. If she doesn't, she's likely to turn in earlier than most people, or to at least grab a power nap. But she sleeps less than most. She's up with the sun. A hearty breakfast with salted eggs and bacon or sausage has her going again. The adrenals speed up the metabolism to deal with stress, and most cholerics can eat a lot without gaining weight. They usually take on demanding work, managing lots of people, high on stress.

But eventually the adrenals can become exhausted, or the choleric humor is dissipated, and the person will start to rely on other humors to get through a demanding day. The choleric person on a salty, red meat dietary plan can burn out before his time. The metabolism slows down and no longer responds to salt and red meat, and the digestion becomes poor because the stress reaction suppresses it repeatedly. So the choleric person begins to experience digestive problems, heartburn, reflux, and/or gastrointestinal problems and is told to change his diet. He begins stimulating secondary humors by eating different stimulating foods.

In fact, no matter what your dominant humor, once it is depleted, and any subordinate humor is also exhausted, sugar eventually becomes the universal craving, because it stimulates the melancholic humor. It sends the depressed system into a manic phase for a couple of hours. It supplies sugar directly to the cellular furnaces, so they get a jolt and the person feels stimulated and effective again for a time. This is the innate pattern of the melancholic, of whom we'll speak in a moment.

Gordon was a choleric gentleman whose dominating nature was out of control. He did everything on a grand scale. His business was very successful and he could give his family anything they wanted. But his wife was tired of him always being away on business trips and didn't like his commanding style with the kids. He had always been big of build, so he didn't think his girth was a problem.

I suggested that dietary adjustments might help balance his choleric humor a bit. His successful business was pushing him hard, and his choleric humor was overstimulated. It was clear he was eating at least two megameals a day, entertaining business contacts, new hirees, and customers. A cocktail and a hearty meat dish seemed always most appropriate to make the guests feel comfortable ordering generously.

We role-played things to say. "I had a grand meal last night, so I'm going light, but you go ahead, order the house." As soon as Gordon lightened up on his adrenal-kicking diet, his mood lightened up too and his phlegmatic wife felt like his interest in the family had returned.

Here's the dietary guidelines he followed for the more balanced choleric.

- Red meat no more than 3 or 4 times a week
- White fish or chicken other meals
- A light breakfast, including fruit or grains
- More salads with the protein meals
- No extra hamburgers or other meals
- No salty snacks or chips
- Snack on vegetables or peanuts or seeds only lightly salted or raw
- Supplement with vitamins C and B-1 and B-2, along with trace minerals from kelp
- Get 7 to 8 hours sleep regularly.

The Melancholic Metabolism

FROM THE POINT of view of the ancients, the melancholic humor is associated with the earth. Sugar provides the basic fuel for metabolism. It is produced by plants from the earth with the help of the energy of the sun during the day. All sugar is converted to glucose in the body by the liver. The mercurial nature of the melancholic apparently comes from the sensitivity of the body to this input of earthy energy.

The typical energy pattern of the melancholic is to crave sugar every two hours or so. That's how long it takes for the sugar to have its manic effect and then subside, as the body works furiously to bring the blood sugar levels back to normal so the cells can rely on normal blood levels of nutrients and electrolytes. In the ancient understanding of the elements, the earth is cold and dry. Plant foods are much more cooling than the red meat the choleric craves. And concentrated sugars have a drying effect similar to salt. Water is pulled from the cells to help dilute the blood, which is overwhelmed by a sudden intake of sugar. Caffeine and chocolate, related substances that stimulate energy production, are also diuretics, causing the body to become more dry. It is noteworthy that just as earth moves little on its own but moves in response to outside conditions like weather, water, wind, and warmth, so those dominated by the melancholic humor are the most reactive to changes in these outside conditions.

From the scientific point of view, the ancient recognition of the melancholic person's tendency to drug herself with sweets can be attributable to the action of the thyroid gland. The body has a very sophisticated mechanism for maintaining the concentration of glucose in the blood. Sugar is extremely drying and if the concentration becomes too high in the arteries on the way from the intestines or the liver to the cellular tissues, the cells that line the arteries get dehydrated and lose their resistance to injury by all the materials flowing by. Eventually proteins, minerals like calcium, and fats, including cholesterol, stick and patch the injured parts, but if the situation is not reversed, the body develops arterial diseases of hardening and dangerous plaque blockages. These problems are not restricted to melancholics because, as mentioned before, all types of temperaments come to crave the sugars and refined carbohydrates that cause these problems if they remain out of balance over time.

To protect the flow of necessary oxygen and nutrients—namely the amino acids for protein, the fatty acids for fats, and vitamins and minerals—to all the cells by way of the blood system, your body is very careful to regulate sugar content.

This means that when you eat sugar in a concentrated form so that it increases blood sugar dramatically, the body has a mechanism by which the pancreas releases insulin. Insulin quickly influences the cells to pull sugar from the blood. Problem is, the tissue cells will get dehydrated by this sudden influx of sugar just like the arterial cells. So the thyroid gland produces hormones that quickly speed up the cellular metabolism to burn up the sugar fast to form oxygen and water, so that the sugar will not destroy the cells.

The sudden energy surge the melancholic person experiences is from this sudden thyroid dependent increase in metabolism. But it lasts only about ninety minutes. Then she needs more sugar to keep up the energy level or she will go for the caffeine family of substances that have a similar effect to the thyroid hormone in turning up the cellular furnaces. Melancholics like coffee, are usually the chocoholics in any group, and also go for Pepsi over Coke (a sweeter flavor than Coke, and don't think Pepsi doesn't know it!).

If your melancholic friend avoids sugar, she may instead focus on starches, like breads, bagels, cereals, pastas, and muffins. Melancholics love the low-fat diets because they prefer the starchy foods anyhow. The sugary breakfast cereals touted as the great American breakfast for kids today gets them off to an early start for hyperstimulating their thyroid glands and melancholic moods. It's an ideal situation for the food processors whose greatest profits come from cheap, long-lasting, starchy, sugary, flavored, and colored thyroid-addicting foods.

Fat does not come from the earth the way starches do, by way of plants. Fats come from animals or from seeds that plants lift high above the earth to be carried away by wind, water, and animals. Melancholics need quality fat and must focus on the non-carb vegetable foods, or foods with a low glycemic index—that is, they are not metabolized quickly into blood glucose and so don't stimulate the insulin response. Melancholics are the first people in a group to opt for vegetarianism—just the opposite of cholerics, who hardly ever consider it unless forced by their health adviser.

Beer and wine are even more concentrated stimulants to the melancholic humor than sugar alone. They are fermented from starch and the body converts them for energy use. They stimulate the insulin-thyroid process like sugar. Melancholics usually prefer them to distilled spirits because they still contain some carbohydrate, and so give the melancholic the sweet taste they adore.

The melancholic who is keeping his mood or energy up by indulging in a high-carbohydrate diet will tend to exhaust the thyroid over time. Thyroid problems are incidentally at a new high as a result of the low-fat, high-carb diet recommendations that were made toward the end of the last century in efforts to reduce blood fats. Unfortunately, this advice is misguided, since blood fats are most quickly produced in excess not from dietary fat but by carbohydrates, again in the body's effort to protect the blood from dramatic fluctuations in blood sugar content.

Much of these negative consequences of carbohydrates can be overcome by learning about the glycemic index of foods, that is, their tendency to cause the production of insulin in the pancreas, which in turn stimulates the thyroid to build hormones, which speed up the metabolism to burn the sugar that the insulin has pulled into the cells. Hypoglycemia and prediabetic conditions can be avoided. Melancholics may feel deprived on a low-carb diet, but if they stick with melons, grapefruit, berries, and tropical fruits, as well as rye and oats, avoiding white breads and refined sugars and highly fermentable fruits, they can still enjoy the sweet tastes they love.

In any case, the melancholics have been particularly misled by the high-carb recommendations of recent years. They are experiencing an all-time high in allergies, depression, and fatigue. After sugar no longer is enough to get the thyroid going and to give the energy boost the melancholic dominant person is used to, she becomes quite susceptible to caffeine addiction or even alcohol addiction. They far outnumber other groups too in classes on weight loss and nutrition because they have difficulty staying with a low-calorie diet when their energy levels slip so fast.

Frequent consumption of sugar and starches also taxes the metabolic powers of the body so that vitamins and minerals missing from processed foods are soon depleted and any number of metabolic imbalances can follow.

The more this person of the melancholic temperament indulges the sugar/caffeine cycle, the more exaggerated become her melancholic characteristics, until the humor is depleted completely. At that point, depression may become clinical and dangerous, and the melancholic may be subjected to psychiatric drugs, rather than the dietary changes that would allow the body to reestablish humoral balance.

The oversensitive thyroid gland of the melancholic can be under- or overactive at different stages of life. The thyroid hormones tend to stimulate the parasympathetic nervous system that causes expansion of the body's systems, for relaxation and creating a more outgoing, creative feeling.

The melancholic can be animated and talkative at one minute and nodding off the next. The blood sugar roller coaster he is on can run his life. These people may pass out after dinner or stay up all night depending on their shifting moods. They crave long lazy mornings in bed but often sleep poorly on a normal night because of big variations in blood sugar levels, especially in the early-morning hours when liver stores of the glycogen form of glucose are depleted and blood sugar levels sink.

Muffins or bagels in the morning, the classic urban breakfast, or skipping breakfast in an effort to lose weight, both put the melancholic right back into the sugar-stimulant up and down cycle. Watch in the typical office setting how many people must have coffee, chocolate, or a starchy snack every two hours or so. It is a national phenomenon!

Those of the melancholic temperament often fall asleep after meals because of the drop in blood sugar brought on by the insulin overresponse to too much carbohydrate in the meal. If you want to stay awake, have protein foods with salad and skip the starches and dessert.

Many people who are trying to diet fall into the melancholic category. Just as they are sensitive to the weather, they are sensitive to their own weight and shape. Because of their tendency to mercurial moods, mood-stimulated eating is especially common with them.

Sandy was just such a person. She loved her work designing fashion displays for department stores, but she was embarrassed to be around the glamorous perfume people, makeup artists, and occasional models at the stores. She wanted to be able to show off her long legs again and reduce her cup size a little, as well as reduce her large upper arms. She had had some success with some popular diet programs, which are usually designed for the melancholics, but as a melancholic, she didn't like the limits on her freedom and the constant record keeping and accountability the diets required. Also, her moodiness didn't go away.

In the first two weeks of the melancholic diet, she discovered her energy level and moods were more reliable than she could ever remember and she lost weight quickly. Because she felt the diet was working with her instead of against her natural inclinations, she stuck with it when she attained her goals, and was happy to feel beautiful and happy again, both at the same time.

She followed these simple guidelines for melancholics:

♦ Eat a breakfast rich in protein and fat within an hour of arising
♦ Don't snack on carbohydrates
♦ Don't eat anything after 8 at night
♦ Go light on wines, beers, pasta, bagels, and other pure carbohydrates
♦ Eat some protein with each serving of carbs
♦ Drink lots of water and eat salads daily
♦ Prefer quality fats over carbs for energy, like butter, olive oil, nuts and seeds
♦ Supplement with magnesium, amino acids, especially L-glutamine
♦ Don't wait until weekends to get some sleep; turn in earlier

The Sanguine Metabolism

FROM THE POINT of view of the ancient experts, the sanguine humor is linked to the natural element of air, which is carried in the blood, hence the name "sang," the Latin word root meaning blood. The ancient observers could tell from a wound that the blood has a special relationship with air. For one thing, it turns red as soon as it contacts air. For another, people expire, that is, lose their breath, when they lose blood. In most ancient traditions including the ancient Mediterranean, the breath was associated with the spirit. The heart where the blood resided was also the seat of the spirit. Hot-blooded still means passionate and ready to go. The sanguine person is like that.

In the process of sexual arousal, pursuit, and consummation, the blood runs faster, the breathing rate increases, the whole body prepares for an important spurt of activity. Also the blood and air are channeled in particular to the organs of sexual response for maximum comfort and enjoyment and effectiveness of the reproductive and romantic pair-bonding act.

The sanguine dominant person tends toward passion, flow, and interaction, because this humor links to our sexuality. The direct link to current connotations of the word "sanguine" may not be immediately apparent. But I suppose that air and wind flow freely and have their impact only by affecting other substances and elements. The connotation of the sanguine as someone who has a rather serene and optimistic view of life certainly can be associated with a sexual confidence and high level of generous, healthy libido that spills over into a positive attitude toward people and relationships in general.

In any case, sanguines tend to go after aphrodisiac foods like shellfish and pumpkin pie, spices, creams, and dark chocolates. In humans sexual activity tends to occur in the evening and this is when sanguines are generally most lively and most sanguine. They tend to have a pretty reliable output of energy through the day, but enjoy evenings in particular and like to get a regular eight hours sleep, preferably after a romantic interlude.

From the scientific point of view, the sanguine tends to choose foods that stimulate the sex glands, such as spices, shellfish, and creamy fats. These foods are known aphrodisiacs and when the sanguine feels any kind of stress or lag in energy, it is the sex glands that turn up the metabolism under the influence of this humor.

The sex glands, like the adrenals, tend to stimulate the sympathetic nervous system and create contraction in the muscles and organs of the body, preparing the body for the buildup of tension required for sexual release. Sanguines learn early in life that the aphrodisiac foods give them extra energy under stress.

Sanguines like breakfast, but only if it includes eggs—for the creamy fat included in them (cholesterol, saturated fats and phospholipids)—spicy meats like sausage or bacon, creamy fat like rich yogurt or cream-filled pastries, buttery croissants, or cinnamon rolls. Bagels only pass if covered with cream cheese. Unfortunately such a breakfast stimulates the gonadal hormones too early in the day and the sanguine's appetite may be excessive all day after such a meal, or other sanguine traits may be exaggerated.

You may have been thinking that this is exactly the breakfast we are supposed to avoid anyhow, so high in fat and cholesterol. But to help balance the sanguine humor this meal in moderate portions can be quite useful and to a sanguine tastes like heaven if not overdone. As long as the food is farm fresh and free of agricultural and food-processing chemicals and balanced with other humorally sustaining foods during the day, like fruits and vegetables, particularly onions and minimally refined grain foods, it can do no harm to anyone. In fact it has been a mainstay meal of generations of healthy farmers. Only the sanguine and choleric need to take care that a breakfast of this kind is not overdone, because it can overstimulate their humors and exaggerate their traits all day.

The sanguine metabolism is effective at processing fat and so is highly efficient. Sanguines need few calories to have energy. They can put on weight easily but rarely become obese, though they find it hard to take it off. The most frequent problems that arise are related, as with the choleric, to a switch to sugar as the sanguine force gets exhausted, and he starts to go for sugar to stimulate the thyroid, through the melancholic humor. Of course, excessive consumption of refined processed fats—especially hydrogenated oils, stale cholesterol products, and creamy tasting substitutes for real fresh cream and eggs—can lead to major burdens on the sanguine body, especially in the circulatory system.

Patrick will serve nicely as an example of a dietary challenge for a sanguine temperament. As mentioned in the Introduction, he had a promising career but was low on energy because he had been trying to lose weight for over twenty years on all kinds of diets and his self-esteem had suffered because he could not make this one obvious improvement. He marveled that he showed up in the sanguine category. He had never been able, in various typologies he had tried before, to find a profile that matched him. So he had tried low-calorie diets, low-fat diets, grapefruit diet, high-protein diets, and more. Now, though, he had total success and was free of cravings and energy drops, with a diet that included all the elements best for sanguines:

- Small breakfast, no spices, light on natural fats
- No snacking on fatty or creamy foods, chips, and dips
- Snacks of crunchy vegetables or seeds
- No eating after 7 at night
- No fried or hydrogenated fats
- Watch quantities when mixing fat and carbohydrates, as in Italian food
- Lots of salads with quality olive oil and cider vinegar
- Supplement with B-6, vitamins E and A, magnesium, and potassium
- Don't stay up late more than one night at a time

The Phlegmatic Metabolism

IN THE ANCIENT writings, the phlegmatic humor is associated with the element of water. The phlegmatic force or vapor has an affinity for foods that are cool and wet and promote those conditions in the body. The phlegmatic humor is attracted to beverages, fruit juices, milk, and mild soups but not too hot. The most concentrated form of what phlegmatics crave is cheese or cottage cheese, or dairy products sweetened with fruit or sugars. People of the phlegmatic humor often manifest colds and runny noses but usually recover quickly, at least in their younger years. But more about that later.

From the scientific perspective, the phlegmatic humor is all about conserving energy by means of the pituitary gland. This gland tends to channel energy into growth rather than action or even thought. The young calf is expected to be mature and be ready to migrate with its herd in three months, since cattle were designed to roam and graze almost incessantly and move seasonally with the weather. Cow's milk is therefore high in pituitary hormones, the hormones of growth. Humans, on the other hand, stay put or migrate slowly, and even more important, the young are carried for at least four years. We have no need for quick physical growth. Learning and mental development is more important to our species.

Phlegmatic children quickly discover their affinity for milk, if it is offered to them. Unfortunately, it overfeeds their dominant phlegmatic humor. And since the pituitary influence conserves energy, these folks have a hard time staying slim. Being small and efficient at storing fat, they must eat perhaps the least of any of the humors to maintain their figures, especially if they are indulging their phlegmatic humor with sweetened cow's milk products.

It should be noted that though eggs are usually included in the category of dairy products, the phlegmatic person usually actively dislikes eggs while loving milk. So if you ask a phlegmatic person if they like dairy, they may say no, because they don't like eggs. If you ask more specifically, they will agree they like cheese and yogurt. Of all the humoral types, they are the least likely to be aware of what they eat on a regular basis. They think more in terms of occasional snacks.

Yet protein and high-quality fat can do wonders to energize and speed up the metabolism of the phlegmatic, and eggs are a good source of these things. If you have a phlegmatic child, it's worth it to find a form of eggs she likes. A milkshake with an egg yolk thrown in is one possibility. Also, though often lacto-vegetarian (but not ovo-vegetarian), phlegmatic-dominant people do much better if they eat a bit of red meat or at least chicken or other fowl weekly.

For someone of the phlegmatic temperament, the metabolism is slow. It's hard for her to lose weight. She will usually try to lose weight on cottage cheese and fruit—the sweet dairy program. She quickly becomes fatigued and lethargic, though, exaggerating her phlegmatic personality traits. The phlegmatic element, water, goes with the flow, seeks its own level, is flexible and responsive, but immovable once it takes a position. Phlegmatics tend to be a lot like that.

Milk bears a strange resemblance to thick mucus, I hate to say, especially the homogenized, pasteurized, denatured milk that most phlegmatics are stuck with in today's marketplace. Fresh milk is actually much sweeter, and if this were widely available phlegmatics might not be so drawn to sweets and might be satisfied with less milk. Likewise today's milk has fat that is severely modified by the homogenization process or just simply removed from fat-reduced milk like buttermilk, skim, or 2 percent milk. This means that even milk today is a fractionated, overprocessed food and cannot support a healthy body.

It has been known for centuries that milk can be mucus-forming for some people. Many societies use only fermented milk products if they cannot consume the milk immediately after being taken from the mother animal. This processing by other organisms renders the milk less mucus-forming in the human gut by starting digestion and adding enzymes. Children who drink a lot of milk often avoid greens because the milk has formed excess mucus in the digestive system and greens have the opposite effect—a tendency to clean and sweep out mucus, thus creating an uncomfortable conflict most people including children will try to avoid. When parents cut down on the milk they serve their children, they often find their children much more willing to begin eating their vegetables.

So dramatic is this phenomenon that when parents have asked me why they cannot get their children to eat vegetables, I immediately offer a guess that the children are big milk drinkers and am regularly on target with my guess. One must be careful, however, with such questions, because parents in this society often think that one glass per meal does not make for a big milk drinker, although by traditional standards it does.

People with sluggish metabolisms have long been known to benefit from a higher protein diet, especially in fish and organ meats, lots of vegetables, and minimal dairy.

From the scientific point of view, the phlegmatic humor corresponds to the pituitary gland, which produces a number of hormones that regulate other glands and especially the human growth hormone. One reason children need lots of sleep is because this hormone is primarily replenished during sleep. You can see how this hormone provides the chemical explanation for why infants grow so fast. Pituitary production of HGH is highest in infancy.

Pituitary hormones tend to have a stimulating effect on the parasympathetic aspects of the body, expansive for the melancholic, relaxing and comforting for the phlegmatic.

It may be interesting to note that the consumption of milk by children in the developed countries has been associated with larger development and earlier maturity than in other cultures or previously in our own. Again, phlegmatics tend to stay more youthful and childlike than most, well into their adult years. But their libido tends to be weak. Perhaps their body continues to think it is in a growing mode rather than a reproducing mode?

Phlegmatics are the least likely to drink alcoholic beverages, and if they do, being agreeable people, they will prefer the milder, sweeter drinks, like light beers or wine coolers or sangria. They are easily inebriated.

For the phlegmatic temperament, you might want to meet Brenda. She was petite and youthful and loved helping people. Thing is, she wasn't going out much anymore because she was upset about how round she was getting, especially since she had her children. She was also developing some serious fatigue around her workday. She knew she could lose weight on a cottage cheese and fruit diet, but the pounds always came back when she got tired and run-down and went off the diet.

Brenda was relieved to learn she was a phlegmatic. It was confusing at first, because she had followed popular advice about consuming lots of milk in pregnancy for the baby and then lots of milk for mature women to support the bones. But we reviewed how effective the body is in balancing calcium and other minerals so long as there are good sources in the body, and how exercise, which phlegmatics often avoid because of fatigue, helps keep the bones mineralized if you have a good source of minerals from vegetables and soups and whole grains, along with some meat.

The changes took some time to make, but she made steady progress toward her goal over the next few months and regained enough energy to start a rewarding walking regimen with a neighbor. She followed this simple advice for phlegmatics:

- Have a breakfast with some kind of protein and minimal milk
- Have a regular lunch, again with protein, perhaps chicken, fish, or pork
- Have a salad a day with lots of colorful vegetables like peppers and tomatoes
- Use high-quality fats, such as olive oil or pumpkin seeds, in moderation
- No milk or cheese for snacks; only at meals
- Snack on vegetables, peanut butter, and crackers
- No milk or cereal at bedtime
- Supplement with chlorophyll, vitamin D, and trace minerals
- Get lots of sleep but start the day early

As you may have gathered from the descriptions of tastes and preferences by humor, the humors cause you to be attracted to the highly concentrated prepared foods that most stimulate your dominant or sometimes subdominant gland. If you are ignorant of how imbalancing these can be, you are likely to indulge the attraction. At the same time, many people have heard that a child left to pick his own food from a smorgasbord of choices will pick a balanced diet over a period of time such as a week. This is indeed the case, but only if the foods are not overprocessed. If the flavors are not concentrated and micronutrients not depleted so as to fool the child's inner guidance system, the child's tastes will not be distorted but will tell the truth of what's good for health. In the studies referred to in these reports, the foods were relatively unprocessed. The purpose of the study was to see if children chose from the various food groups to balance protein, fats, vitamins, and minerals. It was not designed to test whether humoral cravings would win out against natural instincts in the wild. They will and do all the time.

For parents the clear message is, put good quality unprocessed foods before your children and then you don't have to worry so much about whether they eat an exact balance of nutrients at each meal. They will naturally tend to do so. Then be aware of their temperaments if any undesirable traits of health or character appear.

So humoral cravings can lead us astray in a number of ways once our foods have been processed in a manner that caters directly to our humoral stimulators. And don't think for a minute that the food processing industry doesn't know that the great triggers to compulsive eating are overconcentrated sugars, starches, red meat, milk, salt, creams, and spices.

In the material that follows, we will build on the basic recommendations you have heard here so that you can bring yourself back into balance and still enjoy the occasional treat, even to suit your humor, without going overboard and without feeling guilty or out of control. This kind of comfortable eating is done without medicine, drugs, or any expert services. Rather, by understanding your own balance of humors, you can achieve total dietary freedom. That's saying something when you consider how far out of balance you can get with the ready availability of concentrated refined processed "foods" everywhere. They are really drugs, defined as prepared substances designed to have a specific metabolic effect rather than for general nourishment. Like drugs, refined foods are designed for a specific purpose—to stimulate glands, produce extra energy, or create allergic or stress responses for a temporary sense of well-being. They are not designed to nourish the body as a whole, and empower the body/mind itself to decide how to balance all the forces at work.

Or, in the ancient humoral language, you could say that these severely altered foods are designed to directly manipulate the humoral flow of vital forces, often to your detriment, instead of supporting a regular nourishment of the whole body to allow for dynamic and flexible adjustment and rebalancing of the humors for the greatest well-being of the whole organism—that is, you.

Now that you have heard about the eating choices associated with the different humoral temperaments, please take a look at Figures 22 and 23 for a review.

Then you can spend some time taking in all the information in Figure 25. This chart is designed to bring together a number of different aspects of physique, temperament, energy usage, dietary tendencies, and recommended dietary changes. Some of these are further illustrated by the more whimsical depictions of each humor in Figure 24.

The key to balancing your humors with diet is to focus first on complete nourishment, then avoid in particular those refined foods that overstimulate your dominant gland, and emphasize those foods that nurture all the glands and gently nudge the less active ones. You might refer again here back to the ten points listed in Chapter 1.

Once you have assimilated this valuable information about yourself and those around you who form a part of your life, you can begin to design ways to use diet and other factors to move yourself to better humoral balance, a happier temperament, and a more fulfilling life.

One point of caution. While you are responsibly avoiding junk foods that can overstimulate your dominant gland, you may be tempted to shore up subordinate humors with the fast foods that stimulate them. For example, if you are a melancholic and know you should avoid carbs for snacks, you may think salty chips will be all right. While they will do less to exaggerate your melancholic humor than a sugary soda and will give a kick to your adrenal and sex glands, your choleric and sanguine aspects, they still will not give your body what it needs to restore and maintain humoral health. Instead, if there are any challenges in your life, in any area, take care to minimize junk foods of any kind. Seek foods that actually nourish your dominant humor rather than overstimulate your other humors, and also seek foods that gently favor and nourish your subordinate glands rather than over-stimulate them.

Many of my students and clients over the years have used a standard for quality foods that I developed for my own family to help gauge how far we had strayed into the field of overprocessed foods. This standard for quality I call "Wolfspring." It is an acronym that is easy to remember and can be used to check the different dishes you

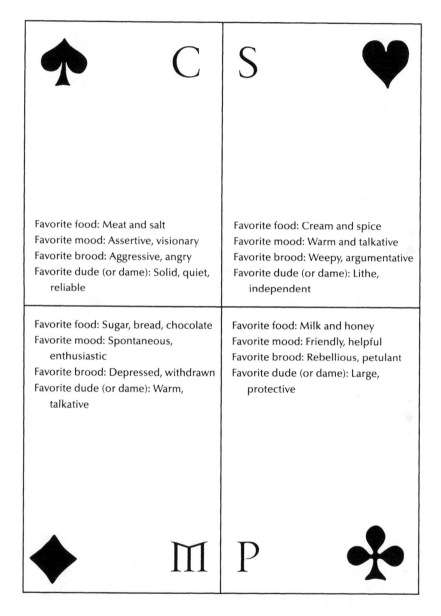

FIGURE 24. The Whimsical Humors. Here's another opportunity to play with the humors and imagine the corresponding temperaments. This time the clusters cut across all the different aspects of health, personality, and character that we have been examining. Favorite brood refers to what these people do when they are feeling bad and out of humor.

HUMOROLOGY - SUMMARY CHART OF KEY TENDENCIES

Humor	Ancient Element/Season	Dominant Gland	Ancient Character	Strongest Cravings
Choleric	fire-summer	adrenal	hot-dry	meat-salt
Sanguine	air-spring	gonadal	hot-moist	fats-spice
Melancholic	earth-fall	thyroid	cool-dry	carbs-caffeine
Phlegmatic	water-winter	pituitary	cool-moist	dairy-sugar

Humor	Protein/Fat Metabolism	Physical Character	Best Mood	Worst Mood
Choleric	strong	square build fat above waist	decisive vigorous	angry aggressive
Sanguine	strong	curvy build fat below waist	passionate patient	bombastic weepy
Melancholic	weak	slight build fat at middle	creative enthused	depressed withdrawn
Phlegmatic	weak	rounded build fat all over even	dedicated supportive	rebellious lethargic

FIGURE 25. **Humorology: Summary Chart of Key Tendencies.** This is a chart I have used in hundreds of workshops and private sessions. The profiles and characteristics described here are merely tendencies and statistical predictions. They may not be so, or prove true in any specific case. In few cases will they all hold true. A cluster is usually evident to an experienced, clinical humorologist and will serve for predicting and recommending dietary behavior and related health factors. The purpose is to maximize the innate potential of each individual for total health and balance by sound holistic guidance in lifestyle choices. Tolerance and "humor" are essential.

Humor	Oxidation Rate	Favorite Meal	Happiest Profession	Carbohydrate Metabolism
Choleric	fast	dinner	manager-statesman	strong
Sanguine	slow	breakfast	teacher-communicator	weak
Melancholic	fast	lunch	artist-theorist	strong
Phlegmatic	slow	snack	craftsperson- helper	weak

Humor	Snack-time Urge	Facial Features	Balancing Diet
Choleric	early eve.	large, square	small, carb-based breakfast, meat just once a day
Sanguine	late eve.	small, heart	small, low-fat breakfast, no snack after dinner
Melancholic	any time	large, oval	protein breakfast, smaller dinner, no sugar snacks
Phlegmatic	mid-afternoon	med., rounded	protein breakfast, dairy just once a day, no dairy snacks

♠ C	S ♥
dry and warm To rebalance after a hot tennis game, try a cool glass of water or a leisurely swim Beware of overdoing it in the summer	moist and warm To rebalance after a warm shower, spend a moment with the water turned cool Take care not to take on too many projects in the spring, be selective
dry and cool To rebalance after a cold winter day, have a warm cup of soup or a warm bath As fall approaches, take special care to support your immune system and stay positive	moist and cool To rebalance after a busy day of errands, have some saltines or sit a while in the sun In winter, take care to stay warm and avoid too many beverages or long baths
♦ ⅲ	P ♣

FIGURE 26. **Elemental Qualities and Environmental Influences.** Simple as it may seem, some very elementary changes of environment in accordance with humoral correspondences can help prevent ailments to which particular temperaments may be prone.

are serving yourself and your family for overall quality and compatibility with the healthy processes of the body. WOLFSPRING stands for: Whole (not overly refined), Organic (grown without pesticides, etc.), Local (in harmony with local conditions), Fresh, Simple (not a challenge to the digestive system), Pure (not processed with a lot of additives and preservatives), Raw (for foods that are safe raw), In season (more compatible with other conditions you are experiencing), Not irradiated, and Genetically traditional.

The further you depart from these qualities in your basic food patterns, the more likely it is that you are eating foods that will negatively impact your temperament. It is no accident that the temperaments are coming to the fore again, I believe, now that refined foods have become the rule rather than the exception. The Hippocratic doctors treated the wealthy classes who could afford the labor necessary to refine their foods and create delicacies for the palate. As a result, these patients suffered many of the degenerative conditions we are experiencing now. But for us, their incidence is not limited to the wealthy. In fact, they are more prevalent among the poor in an ironic reversal since ancient times. With refined foods being cheaper than whole foods as a result of modern technology and chemistry, the wealthy are drawn to healthier whole and naturally prepared foods, while the less wealthy accumulate degenerative imbalances as a result of overprocessed foods.

When the population's habits of life are significantly distorted, the temperaments are more dramatically exaggerated, and people start to notice again the effects of bad humor in the people around them. It will take concerted effort to get ourselves educated enough about these matters to get our health back as a society. Again it is no accident that more than half of our population is overweight. We are out of balance, out of humor, and in bad temper.

It is sad but true that irradiation and genetic engineering were hardly heard of when I originally put them into the WOLFSPRING standard. Now they are front page news. I urge you to take action to assure a safe, balanced, and balance-creating food supply for yourself and those you love.

Meanwhile, if you feel your life is out of balance and your humors are pulling you in directions you don't want to go, make a check of your diet and make the changes necessary for the results you want. You may be amazed at the difference.

In the next chapter, you will see why it can be so important to know your humors even if you have no serious complaints at this time. Ben Franklin said that an ounce of prevention is worth a pound of cure. The lifestyle suggestions you have just heard can form the basis of a preventive approach to health. In the next chapter, you will learn about the specific disease tendencies of the four temperaments. Then in the chapter following, you will find out more about what changes and adjustments you can make to prevent or overcome many disease conditions, even if they have gained a foothold in your life.

Adequate nutrition is influenced by endocrine patterns, that is by the make-up of our particular mechanism or machine. Our endocrine patterns are inherited and certain physical characteristics indicate general nutritional needs. We all require carbohydrates, proteins, fats, vitamins and minerals. All of these elements are necessary to everyone, but because of physical differences, the quantities vary for each individual. . . .

The means of estimating the dietary needs of each individual are twofold:

First, physical characteristics indicate ancestry. In the past, people in general did not move about much; they lived and died in the same place and their children and children's children after them. As the generations went on, their physical beings were modified by their particular environment. Nutrition, an important part of their environment, was reflected in their bodily developments. . . .

The second means of determining the dietary needs of each individual are the instincts. . . . It is my belief that a person will not need to consider the number of calories in his diet, the amount of energy foods and so forth if an adequate supply of minerals is provided and devitalized foods are omitted from the diet. . . .

In a state of nature we have four tastes, sweet, sour, salt and bitter. [They] lead us to a variety of foods. In no one of them do we find just one nutritional element; each contains vitamins, proteins and carbohydrates. So when our bodies crave sweet or sour they are demanding not an unadulterated sweet, like sugar, but sweet plus.

—MELVIN E. PAGE, D.D.S., *Degeneration—Regeneration* (1949, 1980), pp. 77–80

Your Humoral Health History:
Disease Patterns by the Humors

... [T]his unguento, this rare extraction, that hath only power to dispense all malignant humours that proceed either of hot, cold, moist, or windy causes ...

—VOLPONE, pretending to have a panacea, in Ben Jonson (1572-1637), *Volpone* (1606), in Dutton, *Ben Jonson: To the First Folio,* II.ii.91–93

HEN THE BODY is healthy and the mind serene, you are at ease. If either is out of balance, you begin to suffer disease. The diseases we worry about today are usually imbalances that have progressed way beyond their first signs, sometimes for decades. With humorology, you can become much more sensitive to the first signs and stop problems before they start. "A stitch in time saves nine," or "an ounce of prevention is worth a pound of cure." Both of these aphorisms are from Benjamin Franklin, one of the fathers of our country who lived to a ripe and vigorous old age.

You may find this chapter the least pleasant chapter in this book. You will be reviewing what can go wrong with the humors out of balance. But it is important to know what signs to be aware of so that problems can be avoided. Also, a person's health history can be used to establish easily which humor is in fact dominant and therefore what health program would be most effective and congenial for them.

Specific patterns of disease and disturbance of mind and mood are associated with each humor in dominance, as you probably have garnered from what you have heard so far. It is not pleasant to predict problems based on a person's innate constitution. But far from a condemnation, this kind of awareness gives you what you need to be able to find the dietary, lifestyle, environmental, relationship, and career adjustments that will keep you at your own personal best, free of disease, and in comfort and delight.

Here is an overview of the disease profile for each temperament, if the dominant humor is allowed to persist out of balance.

Disease Tendencies of the Melancholic Out of Humor

THE MELANCHOLIC DOMINANT person is most prone to acute disease conditions. These include most often infections—colds, flus, tonsillitis, and fungal infections. These also include allergy symptoms, which are acute reactions to foreign substances in the environment, either internal or external to the body.

You may wonder whether this is a direct result of the melancholic humor itself or the indirect result of the lifestyle of sugar and starch and irregular rest that the unguided melancholic may fall into. It is hard to tell, really, and may not matter. A healthy melancholic has usually discovered that he does better with more and regular sleep and a quality protein, fat, and vegetable diet. Meanwhile, an unhealthy one is almost always sleeping poorly or at odd hours and overdoing the refined carbohydrates, whether sugar, chocolates, pasta, bread, beer, or wine.

Though allergies and acute infections may plague the childhood and teen years of a melancholic, they may tend to ameliorate and disappear when she becomes an adult. This does not mean the problems are over. The imbalance goes deeper, resulting most often in gastrointestinal problems, most likely brought on by the changes in acidity of the system from a high-carbohydrate diet. Thyroid problems are common also, as you might imagine. Hypoglycemia and diabetes are common threats to the melancholic.

Alternating constipation and diarrhea are a frequent complaint, frequent headaches occur, as well as joint problems, yeast infections, and perhaps osteoporosis. The cold, dry tendency of the melancholic also shows up in the mental tendency toward depression and withdrawal and physically in sinus problems, bronchial infections, and migraines.

The good news is that none of this needs to happen if she is aware of her humoral tendencies. She does not even have to give

Modern Medicine and the Humors

WITH THE BEGINNING of the industrial age, the humors were taken to many embarrassing extremes in an effort to heal the many new afflictions of humankind due to overcrowding, poor sanitation, inadequate diets, and more. Many of these conditions have been overcome by sanitation and nutrition. Others can be controlled through medications. But still little is known about why "one person's remedy is another person's poison," or how we can best prevent disease.

In recent times, modern chemical analysis of disease and modern treatment with pharmaceuticals and surgery have proven less than a total solution. We are looking more and more at ancient and traditional ways of dealing with health challenges, from acupuncture to aromatherapy, diet to homeopathy, therapeutic touch to magnetics, herbs to prayer.

In Europe, emerging into modernity from centuries of nationalist and religious wars and their resulting diseases and plagues, attempts by psychologists, educators, and naturalists to study human nature, health, and the evolution of character led back to an interest in ancient observation.

But in medical matters physicians have in fact moved away from the humors because of new technologies that allowed for microscopic observation of biological systems, paired with the new ability to manipulate petrochemicals. With the revelations about tiny microbes and chemical reactions on the atomic level, the simplicity of Aristotle's four elements fell to ridicule. Once patent medicines derived from petrochemicals became the fashion because of their powerful pharmacological effects, especially in their ability to kill infectious microbes, the use of food, or hot and cold or wet and dry, to rebalance the body in hopes that health would return on its own seemed hopelessly antiquated and quaint. Medical students were told only of the excesses of humoral medicine, like excessive use of bleeding, leeches, colon cleansing, and other unfamiliar and distasteful methods of humoral medicine. These caused disdain and contempt for the ancient ways, even though these had been used even after the Civil War, and even though some rather extreme and distasteful methods are used today, such as shock treatment and chemotherapy, which may also be considered draconian in future generations.

Meanwhile, in the area of character building, the idea that we are predestined to any particular temperament or character tendencies flies today in the face of the modern focus on freedom and human potential for self-betterment. Inborn temperaments and humoral prescriptions alike were dismissed as "a doting mother's imaginings," "Grandma's home remedies," or "old wives' tales." A male dominance in the hierarchical institutions of the West contributed to a dichotomy between the male-oriented scientific and institutional approach to medicine and the homegrown mother to daughter wisdom of traditional health and character building.

But with the waning of the twentieth century we've taken a new look at both health and character. The microbes we thought we had conquered have developed resistance to our favored poisons, and these poisons are starting to poison us as they accumulate in our environment. Meanwhile, we have discovered that some people are resistant to the germs while others are not. This means that the underlying health of people may be just as important as what microbes they have been exposed to. Building the immune system by having the body in balance through a diet and lifestyle that fits your individual metabolism has suddenly become of interest. A popular movement is demanding that conventional medicine take these factors into account.

At the same time, notions of universal liberation from tradition and widespread standardized education have failed to make everyone homogenous and productive. In fact, treating everyone alike, such as by recommending the same diet, style of learning, career paths, and kinds of relationships for everyone, has not promoted mental health and personal satisfaction as was hoped.

Since 1970, the ecology movement, the women's lib movement, and the New Age movement have shifted our national culture toward intuition, wholism, spirituality, conversation with other cultures and religions, respect for ancient ways, and suspicion of high-tech solutions. The stage is set for renewed study and popular interest in the humors.

up chocolate or sweets or breads, so long as she pays good attention to how to keep her humors in balance and uses these only in moderation and at judicious times of day, as occasional treats. But more about that in the next and final chapter about choosing your humoral lifestyle.

Fall is the cold, dry season of the year by ancient reckonings. Think about the ancient Mediterranean. Fall weather was presumed to come from the cold dry steppes of central Asia. Melancholics usually get their worst symptoms in this season. The molds that come when leaves have fallen and are disintegrating on the ground often give them major allergy symptoms. Being particularly careful during this season can help make for a much more healthy and comfortable winter. Since we tend to live indoors in heated buildings all winter, the dryness of conditions indoors can keep the melancholic sick all winter. Keep yourself warm and hydrated, or take a leisurely tropical vacation in mid-winter to rebalance your basic humoral temperament. And get lots of fresh, moisture-laden air in winter.

Avoid seasonal affective disorder, which afflicts lots of melancholics. This is cabin fever or winter doldrums. Because of their earthiness, melancholics are the most sensitive to the weather. Low-pressure days affect their moods dramatically. If you know this, you can more easily restore your mood when the conditions improve, rather than dwell on your bad day.

Disease Tendencies of the Choleric Out of Humor

THE DISEASE PATTERN of the choleric is a smoldering fire. Cholerics rarely get sick. If they do they try to ignore it. Nothing is allowed to interfere with their drive. They tend to ignore small symptoms and go full steam ahead, their adrenal glands kicking into full gear easily to overcome any temporary physical limitation. They often have symptom-free childhoods, except for occasional broken bones that result from pushing themselves to the limit.

As they reach midlife, however, or even thirty, if they have not found a diet and lifestyle that balances their dominant choleric humor with the others, their adrenals may be burned out and problems can begin. Most often, such people develop dramatic problems. Just about everything about cholerics is huge. They tend to show up as type A personalities. This personality type, the driver person, was early associated with proneness to heart attack when heart attack began to become common just before the middle of the twentieth century. High triglycerides and cholesterol are common, as is weight gain around the upper body, chest, and shoulders, so-called male pattern weight gain. (It's really choleric weight gain.)

Unless the driving choleric learns to slow down, eat more vegetables, quality fats, and less food and hard liquor, the prognosis for a long life is not good. It is extremely important for the choleric to learn to warm up before and cool down after exercise and to nourish the other humors as well as the choleric. Dramatic weight gain and heart stress are frequently the results that the hard-driving choleric temperament produces if she or he does not learn to rebalance.

Disease Tendencies of the Phlegmatic Out of Humor

THE DISEASE PATTERN of the phlegmatic is, like the melancholic, often infectious disease, but more of the slow, chronic kind. Such people often develop asthma, ear infections, and later chronic fatigue, joint discomfort, skin ailments, and kidney or intestinal disorders. They may have had a relatively healthy childhood because of the natural dominance of the pituitary influence in childhood, and may be surprised when problems appear in adulthood.

Respiratory problems can become long-standing, as well as skin problems, since their skin tends to be delicate while their digestion is easily compromised, so that the skin becomes a way for the body to eliminate toxins. Lethargy, fatigue, allergy, headaches, and mild depression are common problems, though they often go undetected for long periods because the phlegmatic is so dedicated to getting her work done, putting others' needs first, and being a dependable part of any work team.

The phlegmatic must be wary of relying on certain conditions once they arise to give them a visible reason to force the issue of taking more rest and recreation. The phlegmatic may have to learn to be more assertive about her own needs and wants along with other lifestyle changes in order to take good care of herself and overcome chronic conditions that would tend to get worse under continuing stress and self-denial. She must often learn to put her own health and peace of mind first, in order to be whole enough to really be helpful to others.

Disease Tendencies of the Sanguine Out of Humor

THE DISEASE PATTERN of the sanguine is less dramatic than the choleric, less acute than the melancholic, and less slow developing than the phlegmatic. These people can suffer a variety of problems, but because of their sanguine nature they tend to minimize them. Problems of adequate oxygenation of tissues crop up because of the importance of air, so muscle and soft tissue problems, neck problems, joint problems, sore hands or feet, and sometimes reproductive problems can appear. Mild allergies in childhood are not unusual. These disappear in adulthood when sex hormones are naturally active, but they may be replaced by yeast infections and excessive weight gravitating to areas below the waist, what is called the female pattern (but is really the sanguine pattern).

Sanguines can develop various cardiovascular problems if their preference for fat leads them to unhealthy fats like hydrogenated fats or overheated fries, or trans fatty acids from overprocessing. Skin problems can arise for the same reason—unhealthy fat being pushed from the body.

Male pattern baldness is common in sanguine men, but it is not a health problem. Digestive problems can arise if fat and carbohydrate are mixed frequently in large quantities in the sanguine diet. If the sanguine is careful to use only high-quality fats in moderation, with a balance of lots of leafy vegetables, health can be maintained.

Other Special Health Situations by the Humors

THE FEMALE MENSTRUAL cycle seems quite sensitive to the humors. Choleric and sanguine women tend to have regular periods, melancholics and phlegmatics irregular ones, the first more frequent and the second less frequent than normal. The melancholic and sanguine are most prone to premenstrual stress syndrome if their humors are not in balance. As you may remember, libido is highly responsive to the humors. Often when the humors are rebalanced, women's cycles and moods become more reliable and agreeable. Also, melancholics and phlegmatics are likely to be more uncomfortable during pregnancy than are choleric and sanguine women. The latter enjoy pregnancy the most of all, perhaps because of the high level of sex hormones needed to support the pregnancy and the increased fluid and warmth that accompanies the pregnancy experience.

As far as the development of cancer, which has become such a scourge since the middle of the twentieth century, just about anyone is vulnerable if their humors are out of balance, though perhaps for different reasons. Cancer cells do best in an acid tissue environment, most notable with the choleric temperament. They also thrive when the immune system is suppressed, most common in the melancholic environment. Cancer cells also take hold more easily when the oxygen supply is low, since cancer cells have a low oxygen need, a condition most common in the sanguine environment. And cancer cells do best when tissue function is sluggish because cancer causing toxins persist, most common in the phlegmatic temperament. Each humor then can contribute to the development of major degenerative conditions like cancer.

The worst news in this book is that our diets and lifestyles have deteriorated to such an extent that just about anyone is vulnerable to attack by cancer or other debilitating, degenerative diseases like heart attack and stroke, diabetes, or arthritis. But the good news is that just about anybody can rebuild health and well-being to optimum vibrancy and balance if the changes are made before the body has completely lost its ability to restore itself.

One sign of severe imbalance is the disease of addiction. Addiction afflicts a person on all levels of being. Anyone whose humors are out of balance can become addicted. The essence of addiction is looking for health and happiness in all the wrong places. As you may have gathered from what you have heard so far, each person's dominant humor can foment cravings for quick fixes. Quick fixes actually only increase the imbalance but are seductive because of the temporary sense of well-being they create.

The out-of-balance choleric dominant person will most likely addict to strong booze—whiskey, vodka, or gin—or to cigars, or to work, to glory and recognition, or to food in major quantities, or to all of the above.

The out-of-balance sanguine will most likely addict to tangy, spicy booze, like brandy, port, sherry, or mixed drinks, or to creamy and spicy foods in excess, or to argumentation and lost causes, or to sexual relations. Smoking usually doesn't appeal. Moderation is the sanguine's theme song, but so is brilliant rationalization. Moderation can go to excess in addiction. The sanguine can exhaust his or her health trying to please everyone and keep the peace.

The out-of-balance melancholic addicts most easily to wine and beer, to sugar and chocolate, and also to coffee and nicotine. Many melancholics, tending toward being artists, also may become addicted to the fumes of paint or other art materials and be seduced by the supposedly creative lifestyles of earlier artists who died of consumption (tuberculosis) or smoking or alcoholism. They can also become addicted to the adoration they feel from passionate sex. They are most likely to be erratic in their addictions, sometimes indulging, sometimes contrite, defending their freedom, seldom predictable.

Out-of-balance phlegmatics may get into cigarettes or light beer and sweet wines, or excessive helping of others at the expense of their own health and sanity. Their loyalty can get them into trouble if they become addicted to an addict who relies on their help.

Of course these are generalizations. It is hoped that understanding these typical clusters of behaviors can help you and your loved ones steer clear of pitfalls common to your temperament and adopt healthy habits that appeal to you for rebalancing your humors.

Consider the seasonal correspondences in Figure 25. The progression of the humors according to season would go from spring, to summer, to fall, to winter, that is, sanguine, choleric, melancholic, and phlegmatic. This is also the way that the digestion presumably works from the humoral point of view, to both separate and combine the humors for good health.

The blood forms from the most valuable nutrients we take in, the bile is a digestive juice that helps assimilate fats and fat-soluble vitamins, the black bile is what's left of digestion and must be eliminated, and the phlegm is present wherever there is unwanted material that may irritate the important membranes of the digestive system. All of these important fluids and functions must go on cooperatively, each in its turn, for you to have total health.

Now let us take a look at the second seven-year period (age 7–14). . . .

Fiery-natured cholerics should be given leaf and stem vegetables, along with watery ones like squash and cucumbers. Such foods are light and do not heat the blood. . . .

Sanguine children, with their light and airy, flighty natures and metabolism, need to be helped to get their roots down to earthy things. They must be fed foods that give the metabolism much to do. . . .

Phlegmatics need to be waked up with the help of every kind of warming spice, sharp-tasting roots, mushrooms, fruits, and fruit salads. One should hold back on milk, substituting instead teas made of various flowers and served with lemon. . . .

Melancholic children also need the blossom element and warming foods to relieve them of the oppressive heavy spirits they derive from too strong a connection with the earth. . . .

Again and again we see that this or that quantity of fats, carbohydrates and proteins is not the criterion to go by, but rather the quality, the formative forces that live in substances as a result of the processes that brought them into being.

—RUDOLF HAUSCHKA, *Nutrition* (1983), pp. 196–97

Your Humoral Balance:
Making Corrections for Health, Romance, and Happiness

With us there was a physician; in all the world there was not another like him for talk of medicines and of surgery, for he was trained in astrology. He skillfully and carefully observed his patient through the astrological hours. . . . He knew the cause of every disease—whether hot, cold, moist, or dry—and how it developed, and of what humour. Indeed, he was the perfect practitioner: the cause and root of the disease determined, at once he gave the sick man his remedy. . . . This physician knew well ancient Aesculapius and Dioscorides, and also Rufus, Hippocrates, Haly and Galen, Serapion, Rhazes, Avicenna, Averroes, Damascenus and Constantine, Bernard, Gatesden, and Gilbertine. His diet was moderate—not too much but that little nourishing and digestible. . . . He held on to that which he gained during a plague. For, in medicine, gold is healthful in drinks; therefore, he especially loved gold.

—Geoffrey Chaucer (c. 1345–1400), "General Prologue,"
in *The Canterbury Tales*, pp. 8–9

W HAT TO DO? The best news in this book is that there are lots of things you can do, oodles and oodles, to help get your humors into a healthy balance, and you don't even need to do them all.

It is popular wisdom today that most people know what they should do for their health, but they just don't do it. They put it off, they make promises for the future, they just don't have the energy today, they just don't feel like it right now. This is because they are out of humor, literally. Once they are back in good humor, they will feel more like doing what works. You can turn a vicious cycle of failure into a progressive cycle of success with something as simple as adjusting the temperature and moisture of your room. Imagine that!

If you want a change, all you have to do is simply do the thing that seems most appropriate to you of all the options you will hear in this chapter, assuming you have been really honest with your-self about what your dominant and secondary humors are. Of course, don't fall into the obvious trap of deciding you are of the humor that would benefit most from the behaviors you crave!

For example, if you are high on sweets, but still in pretty good health, don't decide you're a choleric rather than a melancholic because cholerics don't usually have trouble with sweets. You still may be a melancholic, albeit a lucky one. Likewise, a choleric may decide he's a melancholic because his energy has been down late-ly and he wants to indulge in more meat and exercise. Or a san-guine may decide she's a phlegmatic so that she can spruce up her diet with more cream and spices, inharmonious for her but help-ful to the phlegmatic.

Just as in these examples the individuals mislead themselves in order to indulge their humors, it is sad but true that people who are out of balance believe that their worst behaviors are just what's needed to achieve their goals in a tough situation. The humors can distort our mental powers just as they can distort our physical health. Our strengths become our weaknesses when we are out of balance. We become stubbornly persistent in our behaviors instead of flexible and responsive to our situation. We can go into denial about how we are affecting those around us.

For example, for a choleric, charismatic commanding is the natural way for him to get his way, but when he is out of temper, his commanding presence becomes domineering to those around him and they do not want to cooperate. Yet he will want even more to control the others and will persist in pursuing the least effective avenue to achieving his way.

Similarly, a melancholic can inspire others to accommodate his wishes with his enthusiasm and intelligence. But when out of humor, he will pursue his point doggedly with no room for negotiation and will alienate the people he is trying to persuade. Likewise, a bad tempered phlegmatic will insist on loyalty when it is already too late, and the ill-humored sanguine will make that one last repetitive argument when there is no hope for toleration in the face of his bombastic approach. He chooses the worst way to seek cooperation from the people around him.

But if you have come this far, you are taking what you are learning somewhat seriously and would not be tempted to take these false steps.

Just know that with knowledge of your humors you don't need to give up your favorite things, only keep them in their place: right time of day, right size portions, right preparation processes, and right combinations with other foods. It's not as hard as it sounds if you always keep in mind the simple stuff. Cholerics are hot and dry (love cooked meat and salt), melancholics cold and dry (love cereals, breads, and sugars), phlegmatics, cold and wet (love cold milk and berries), sanguines, hot and wet (love warm creams, buttery pastries, spices).

So now, putting together all you have absorbed so far, we can look at what you can do to dramatically improve your humor, in every sense of the word.

Let's begin with the melancholic humor, since that temperament is the most likely of all the temperaments to be seeking solutions to moods and physical symptoms. They predominate in weight loss classes because they are sensitive about extra weight.

Ways to Rebalance the Melancholic Humor

YOU MOST LIKELY will need to reduce your dietary carbohydrates and achieve better rest if you have any complaints in your life you would like to be rid of.

But first, to address short-term challenges to your health and happiness, the key may be to maintain warmth and hydration, since your humor is cold and dry. This does not mean simply drink more water and wear lots of clothes, though this can be an important start. Some melancholics sweat profusely and may feel too hot to bundle up more. Or they already drink a great deal of water. Like a diabetic they are often thirsty, especially when eating sugar.

In addition to the simpler strategies, you must work with your body to create a deeper internal warmth and hydration. This is done multiple ways. For warmth and hydration, here are some key suggestions:

FOR SHORT-TERM MELANCHOLIC ILLS

[1]   Take a long warm shower. This actually gives a cooling sensation by opening the pores so that toxins may escape and by the cooling evaporation as you dry off. Meanwhile, it gives your body a chance to warm up inside. Hydrating the skin is as important as drinking. Make sure your shower water is filtered so that toxins do not settle on the skin and get absorbed, especially chlorine. A relatively new but very effective strategy is to get a shower head that

puts your water through a magnetic field, which declumps the water molecules and makes them much more moisturizing to the body, skin, and lungs. Avoid the uptake of chlorine in the shower by use of a shower filter. This is especially important for the melancholic dominant person, since inhalants can be particularly threatening to their more delicate immune systems and membrane defenses.

[2] Have a quick little meal of foods pleasing to you but not too junky.

[3] Get lots of time out of doors exposed to direct sunlight but not at peak hours. Melancholics are particularly sensitive to weather shifts. Drops in barometric pressure can affect their moods dramatically. To avoid the mercurial swings, absorb as much good energy from the sun as possible when it's shining. Also get the natural moisture of the outdoor air when possible to avoid both dry overheated interior air in winter and stale overmoist air in warm months.

[4] Plan a tropical vacation in the early winter to balance out the dry cold weather of fall.

[5] Favor cool water over cold or icy water for drinking. This is especially important around mealtime to help with digestion and avoid the shock of cold in your stomach.

[6] Eat lots of succulent varieties of fruits and vegetables, meaning the watery ones, like citrus, melon, and berry and lettuce, tomato, celery, and cabbage. Favor these over starchy and sweeter produce like bananas, apples, and pears, and corn, potatoes, and beans.

[7] Minimize dehydrated foods, like breads, that make you drier and colder. Also avoid foods that dehydrate, like sugar, caffeine, and salty foods. Control your intake of acidifying foods like refined fast foods, which make it harder for the body to detoxify and maintain ideal warmth in the tissues.

[8] If you are melancholic dominant and can have sudden melancholic spells, you need most often a kind of quick

fix for your flagging humor, like a few minutes in the breezy shade out of sun and sweat. If you stay focused on simple environmental actions, like removing a layer of clothing or shoes to cool yourself off, you may quickly get past the mood without resorting to dramatic stimulants.

A big risk for melancholics is that this natural instinct to nudge the dominant humor can lead to major trouble because of the accessibility under the conditions of modern civilization of quick fixes that are unhealthy, especially fast foods and overflavored and -treated drinks. Many melancholics get easily hooked on ice cream for the cold and the dehydrating sugar, or sweetened soda for the same reasons (they are ultimately dehydrating as well as cooling).

If only children learned early to modulate their humors through small changes in environmental conditions, rather than obedience to the constant stream of misleading propaganda on TV about pick-me-up energy foods, we would be a much healthier happier society. It's interesting to note that 60 percent of the kids who committed violent murders in the schools in the last five years were on psychiatric drugs for their moods.

If your melancholic condition seems chronic, then rather than a short-term nudge to your dominant humor, you need to focus on letting it rest and nourishing the other humors, while supporting a balanced flow of your dominant humor. What this means for the melancholic is that if chronic depression or frequent mood swings or digestive or immunological problems persist, you need to do some or all of the following.

FOR CHRONIC MELANCHOLIC CONDITIONS

[1]   Establish a routine through the day for meals, work, play, and sleep. A routine relaxes the frenetic tendencies of the melancholic.

[2]   Eat some of those foods you usually don't. Even if you have been eating wholesome foods, if the downside of the melancholic is showing, you have almost without fail slipped into excessive starch or sweet foods, perhaps whole

grain breads, pastas, or muffins, if not out and out chocolate chip cookies. Now have more lean white fish varieties, organic chicken dishes, with lots of cooked vegetables, warm hearty soups with aduki beans or lentils, rich fresh nuts and seeds, and eggs lightly cooked in lots of butter. Mix sardines with mayonnaise to make a nucleic-acid-rich spread for rye crackers to help rejuvenate all your tissues.

[3] Avoid sweet or starch snacks or bedtime nibbles. Instead eat any carbohydrates in your diet in small portions with meals.

[4] Do something really creative that you've always wanted to do. Perhaps something off by yourself—a greeting card on the PC, your version of a van Gogh landscape or a Calder mobile, singing, dancing, or creative cooking.

[5] Explore ways to express your creativity at work. Invent a new project and be sure you have the freedom to execute it your way.

[6] Throw a party and do your own decorating and catering. Plan out every detail and invite only the people you want.

[7] Choose something you've been wanting to buy, no matter what, and schedule all the time you need, no matter how long, to really shop around and find exactly what you want at the price you want from a favorite store.

[8] Sleep more. Get really comfortable, temperature-wise and moisture-wise. Don't sleep late. Instead go to sleep earlier. And make sure your stomach isn't full of refined snacks at bedtime. A cup of yogurt or a glass of not too cold goat's milk will help you fall asleep quickly. If you eat close to bedtime, you will not only sleep poorly but you will not be hungry for breakfast. And breakfast is a must for melancholics—a protein-rich breakfast.

[9] Engage in vigorous exercise that requires a lot of change of position and change of pace. And explore different kinds of exercise. The melancholic abhors monotony and any threat of boredom. So keep your exercise routine fresh. Above all, have one. The melancholic is very physical—the

earthy type—and if she's not doing physical things she quickly gets too into her head and becomes overwhelmed by the imperfections of her life, other people, the weather, politics, her work, and so on. The physical outlet is crucial to nourishing the earthy melancholic and keeping her in balance.

In summary, indulge the creative and natural physicality of your personality in order to avoid seeking an artificial sense of health through temporary fast food fixes or worse. Meet your tendency to changeability with a routine that you can really look forward to and change it whenever it gets boring. Now let's consider the choleric temperament.

Ways to Rebalance the Choleric Humor

THE CHOLERIC IS a "born leader" even if he doesn't know it, and basically he won't be satisfied until he is leading or spearheading some large enterprise, whether it's a team, a corporation, a family or a community. If the choleric is in good health, and enjoying life in general, but begins to show excessive choleric tendencies, like a domineering tone, or aggressive angry postures, or excessive eating, drinking, or competitiveness at the expense of his own best interests, it's time to notice that an acute situation of imbalance has arisen.

In an acute imbalance, remember, you need to try a nudge to your dominant humor. Chances are it's negative qualities are coming out sideways because it is missing direct opportunities for outlet and expression.

When she wants to lead but doesn't know it or is blocked from doing so in some way, the choleric tries to force obedience through domination and intimidation, which is of course in most cases a quick way to assure that no one actually wants to follow her as their leader.

So what can you do as a choleric if some sudden unpleasant symptoms of imbalance appear?

FOR SHORT-TERM CHOLERIC ILLS

[1] Get physical, not with your challenger, but by entering athletic competition. Play racquetball, golf, tennis, any game that pits your courage, skill, and stamina against that of other champions.

[2] Make sure your breakfast isn't so heavy with meats and salt that your stress response from your adrenal glands—your instinct to fight or fly and your preferred metabolism booster as a choleric—isn't on full tilt all day. Prefer instead a lighter breakfast of an egg or two and oat cereal with a fruit. Cholerics rarely eat fruit until their adrenals are exhausted from thirty years of stress and their thyroid takes over, producing the energy boosts needed to get through the day. But please do it before you have to.

[3] Skip that martini or other hard liquor at the end of the workday. Instead take a power nap. Cholerics often believe they need only five or six hours sleep but after a few decades it catches up with them in their health.

[4] Check your temperature and humidity. Cholerics rarely pay any attention to environmental conditions or even their level of discomfort or pain. Break that habit if you notice unpleasant choleric qualities are showing. A classic story would be a choleric-dominant tennis champion who gets more and more aggressive in a difficult match and ignores his or her level of discomfort from the dry heat as noon approaches, and then suddenly can't continue because of frightening chest pains. Don't go that route. You're already a winner. Take care of yourself before, during, and after the game.

[5] Take a short, warm shower to support your choleric humor gently and elementally so it doesn't tend to show itself in an unpleasantly choleric mood. Or even better, take a gentle sauna, with dry heat. But don't overdo it. The sauna brings blood to the surface and actually helps cool the pent-up heat of the choleric, but too much will backfire.

What if you as a choleric are chronically out of balance? You command and dominate often when you don't need to. You hear rumors about yourself being tough to work with or for. You fall asleep too early in the evening, just when you want to give attention to your family. Or you bring work home and never seem to get to bed. You start to wonder if you might be a workaholic. Perhaps your normal nonstop energy is slowing down. Or your blood pressure stays chronically high.

Any of these chronic conditions means that your humors are in chronic imbalance. You need to get away from temporary solutions for your dominant humor and find deep support for the choleric humor, while nurturing the other humors. Don't let them stay lazy, so to speak, letting the choleric carry all the burden of existence. Here are suggestions for rebalancing the chronically out-of-balance choleric-dominant individual. When symptoms persist, think about what a warm dry powerhouse really needs.

FOR CHRONIC CHOLERIC CONDITIONS

[1]   Eat a modest breakfast that nourishes your other humors and avoids overstimulating the choleric. A hot dry breakfast like a well-cooked omelet and crispy bacon won't do. Go for cooler, wetter dishes, like a bowl of oatmeal with some goat's milk for the phlegmatic humor and perhaps a little cinnamon to awaken the sanguine. Or add some succulent vegetable to your omelet, like sautéed onions, tomatoes, or peppers. Cholerics often avoid vegetables. Vegetables are soft, wet, cooling. This influence doesn't attract the choleric person in her drive to be driven. But if too much of the choleric is showing, it's time to change.

[2]   Get involved in activities where you can't be in a leadership role. Join a bridge foursome and rotate partners. Volunteer in a field where you know you have few skills and will have to be instructed. For example, if you have always worked with your mind and consider yourself a beginner with hammer and nails, volunteer a day a week

at Habitat for Humanity and turn down all the invitations
you will soon get to be supervisor.

[3]   Take a vacation to a cool part of the world, like Alaska. And
don't immediately volunteer for competitive enterprises
like catching the biggest salmon. Instead, take time alone
to examine the scenery, or relax (I know it's a dirty word
with many cholerics) on a short cruise, and see how many
new people you can get to know just to learn about them,
with no thought about how they can further your dreams
or vision, for yourself, them, the cruise line, or the world.

[4]   Get involved with children and reacquaint yourself with
the chaos of newness and spring. For example, get
involved with your children's or grandchildren's art projects (note I did not say coaching their competitive
sports!). Join a children's museum or petting zoo and
volunteer at the gate or one of the rides.

[5]   Plan a romantic evening with your spouse or special
someone and invite them to make all the decisions while
you just carry out their suggestions.

[6]   Spend an hour, or half an hour alone in an art gallery,
museum, or mall and look for beauty and humanity in
whatever your see.

If you do one or more of these things your powerful choleric
constitution will come back into dynamic balance with the other
influences of the humors and your admirable side will reemerge—
your gusto, magnanimity, vision, inspiration, and deeply caring
leadership.

Ways to Rebalance the Sanguine Humor

WHAT IF YOU tend toward a dominant sanguine humor? In an
acute, temporary imbalance, you may tend to get suddenly weepy or
pleading and argumentative without an obvious cause. Perhaps you
feel frustrated that none of the relationships you've been cultivating

recently at home or at work are going the way you would like or meeting your needs. What can you do?

Here are some suggestions for ways to "satisfy" or nudge your sanguine humor gently so that it does not get stuck in the negative mode.

FOR SHORT-TERM SANGUINE ILLS

[1] At your next meal, indulge in something creamy, like rich yogurt, a thick salad dressing, or a fruit compote. Or have some dish with a bit of crunch or spice, like an Indian curry with flat crispbread or a cinnamon apple crunch.

[2] Get some exercise. Get hot and wet with effort and sweat. Sanguines like exercise that engages the mind as well as the body, like martial arts, or dancing routines, anything with patterns and progressions. You may enjoy setting your own goals and standards for performance, competing with yourself instead of with others.

[3] Take a hot shower, and end it with a quick turn to cold. Or in winter, go out back after a hot shower and roll in the snow! Seriously, being a sanguine myself, I've done it with great delight. The quick closing of the pores creates a great sensuous boost to the sanguine. In the shower, don't let it be long, since too much hot and wet could overstimulate the sanguine dimension. For quick effect, let the warm water pound for a minute or two on the back of the neck. This is a major entry point for energy, good and bad, for the sanguine.

[4] Plan that romantic evening you've been hankering for and take your time about it. Let it follow its own rhythm rather than trying to make it perfect.

[5] Set aside ten or fifteen minutes to really feel your emotions around whatever has been bothering you. The sanguine is easily trapped inside her own head and needs to spend regular time acknowledging movements of the heart, because they rule the sanguine, consciously or not.

Now, if you wish, we shall take a look at what to do if negative sanguine characteristics are chronic. Perhaps stress builds up and expecting perfect understanding and cooperation from others becomes a setup for disappointment. You may feel you spend all your time explaining or teaching others how to solve their problems or become better at what they do, with very little appreciation or reward. Perhaps your skin is showing signs of stress, or your digestion, or your hormones related to sex or sleep show signs of imbalance.

Here are some ways to deeply support your sanguine humor while waking up the others to do their part and nourishing them consistently.

FOR CHRONIC SANGUINE CONDITIONS

[1] Get plenty of sleep. Sanguines often come alive at night and find they can get a lot done and be very creative after hours. But then they may get up early too because they don't want to miss any of the action—being all about relationships. So planning adequate sleep is a must. Make sure your sleep environment is comfortable, quiet and dark, with good temperature and humidity, neither too high. Sanguines generally sleep well but may not be sleeping deeply enough to rid themselves of the stress of the day. Consider investing in a quality mattress, which creates a relaxing magnetic field to help you let go quickly of all the complex thoughts sanguines are prone to.

[2] Avoid creamy, spicy foods in the morning. The sanguine humor will get a head start on the day and the other humors will get lazy if these stimulating foods start too early. Avoid the scrumptious cinnamon buns with creamy sugar icing. Save these for a dessert after a quality meal. Instead, have a bowl of oatmeal with goat's milk and a little honey, to wake up and nourish the other humors. Add some sunflower seeds and a pinch of salt to wake up the adrenals.

[3] Avoid snacking on creamy, spicy foods. Steer clear of hot Mexican, Indian, or Szechuan dishes until you know you are again in balance.

[4] Be sure showers are not too warm and keep them short. Enjoy a dry sauna from time to time.

[5] Get involved in outdoor play to stimulate your earthy humor. Spend time alone with nature. Everything need not be experienced in a group! In your physical program include team games as well as individual workouts, so you're not always in the wizard or teacher mode.

[6] Let yourself explore leadership roles as well as mentor/teacher ones. Also, explore crafts and helping roles. Take a night school course in some artistic expression you enjoyed in school, like sculpture or pottery.

[7] Drink cool water in small amounts often. This reduces cravings for fatty, spicy foods, which can overstimulate the hot, wet sanguine humor. Avoid before-dinner flavorful aperitifs and flavorful after-dinner cordials. These will make you want more.

[8] Don't eat after dinner, especially fats. It will likely give you a second wind and keep you going into the night, and then make you hungrier the next day! Sanguine folks are often relieved to find out that others, namely other sanguines, experience this too.

If you take on any of these habits to rebalance your sanguine condition, you will gradually help eliminate tendencies to verbosity, argumentation, bombastic outbursts, bitter sarcasm, or pitiful pleading and will replace these with cheerful communications, great wit, boundless energy, and the mental wizardry, pragmatism, and ingenuity people most admire in you.

Ways to Rebalance the Phlegmatic Humor

ACUTE SYMPTOMS FOR the phlegmatic will be crying, complaining, impatience, often symptoms not characteristic of the normally friendly, reliable, good-natured phlegmatic. Physical symptoms may be colds, stuffy nose, cough, soreness, fatigue, chronic discomfort, and crankiness.

What you will need to rebalance quickly can include any of the following actions.

FOR SHORT-TERM PHLEGMATIC ILLS

[1] A hug. Phlegmatics want recognition, devotion, appreciation. They are not quick to hug people, but enjoy a hug greatly from someone they trust. Ask those close whom you trust to give you some extra time and a hug when you need it.

[2] Since phlegmatic humor is cold and wet, a cool drink will often satisfy. This is one reason it is so easy to hook kids, the original phlegmatics, on cold sodas. And even more so on cold milk, with its high pituitary hormone content. Don't go there. Get a quality water system that makes your water pure and tasty enough that you will want to drink it, poured over a few cubes of ice. Add a lemon or lime wedge to it, or crush a strawberry or banana into it, or both.

[3] Do something physically active to overcome your sluggish tendencies, or if you have been too active for your nature—for example, had a demanding day at work—give yourself permission to relax totally and watch a fun movie. But don't get into the milk and cookies.

[4] Have a snack of yogurt and fruit and make sure your next meal has some quality protein and fat.

[5] Play some of your favorite music and let it make you dance, in your own style.

[6] Get down on the floor and play with your kids, grandchildren, or a pet. Do some serious laughing.

What about chronic problems for the phlegmatic? They may include immunological or allergy problems, fevers, sore muscles and joints, creeping weight gain, or on the mental side, spite, erratic behavior, rebellious attitudes, perverse reactions, and self-pity parties.

Here are some helpful suggestions of ways to deeply nourish your dominant humor while awakening and supporting the other three.

FOR CHRONIC PHLEGMATIC CONDITIONS

[1] Have a real breakfast regularly and keep all your meals regular. Keep snacks small so meals will be welcome. Make breakfast protein-rich. Few phlegmatics like eggs, but if you can learn to make them into a nice custard you will probably like them. You can mix an egg into hot oatmeal to support the phlegmatic humor and never feel that common aversion to eggs. The egg helps stimulate the sanguine humor because of the rich high-quality fats, and a pinch of salt will wake up the adrenals. Some natural bacon or sausage for nonvegetarians is also helpful to the phlegmatic. If vegetarian, add prune or prune juice unsweetened for enriching the blood. Also tomatoes and mushrooms are helpful for the phlegmatic's sluggish metabolism.

[2] Get lots of sleep and keep the timing regular. Phlegmatics need more sleep than most. This will give you more opportunity to cleanse your more lethargic system, and then you can have more energy throughout the day if well rested. This creates a positive feedback loop, in which healthy exertion during the day creates a stronger desire for a good night's sleep and a deeper rest, which makes for a better next day.

[3] Make sure you are cultivating supportive relationships that give you kindness and appreciation as well as lots of opportunities to play and help others. If relationships are not of this kind, do become more assertive about your needs and desires. Some relationships you may want to change, such as those with coworkers who are always asking too much of you. Add new relationships with people who encourage your creative side, your intellect, and your

leadership, as well as your helping and task-based skill mastery.

[4] Begin a routine of regular mild exercise, like walking, jogging, or swimming. Make it lots of fun and do it with people who make you feel important and interesting. Share your ideas with them.

[5] Spend more time indulging your own special pleasures— you know what they are—certain kinds of books, music, art, shows, or home-based hobbies or business.

[6] Stay in touch with family regularly, and let them know you are a leader among them. Plan family events and do things your own way. Ask for help at home and at work. Delegate to others.

[7] Take vacations to warm, dry places like islands and deserts, and play heartily.

Now that you have heard some useful recommendations for achieving a better balance of the humors, so that the best of your natural temperament will emerge, let's review once more the rebalancing strategy.

In an acute situation, do something simple to feed your dominant humor. If you are normally in balance as a sanguine, for example, and you suddenly get weepy, try a cup of hot spicy tea. Give yourself a quick corrective of warm and wet for the sanguine, cold and dry for the melancholic, and so on.

In a situation of chronic imbalance, avoid foods, routines, environments, and even people who encourage your dominant humor. Instead, make lifestyle changes that deeply nourish all your other humors as well as your dominant one. Avoid quick fixes for the other humors as well as for your dominant one. Check your diet and remove the foods that overstimulate your dominant gland and return to natural whole food analogs of those foods you have been craving.

Check when you are eating, as well as what, and check your sleep routine and the amount of heat and moisture in your environment. Refer back to the suggestions of what exact adjustments

to make. It doesn't really matter which ones; that's the beauty of
the humors. You are really dealing with ethereal forces here, not
just this mineral or that vitamin. The body then can use its own
wisdom to get you back on track. Remember, you don't need to
force anything. The humors operate not by force but by flow.

Sharing the humors with family and friends

A FREQUENTLY ASKED question at this juncture is, how do I help
my friends and family? Don't be surprised if some are skeptical.
In the modern era, starting with the industrial revolution and
our ability to harness fire at high temperatures to manipulate
metal, we have been fascinated by the way we can see so much
more and make matter do whatever we want. We have forgotten
how much of life we just can't see, touch, or manipulate to our
will. But with the advent of the twenty-first century, we appear to
be regaining some respect for the unseen and unseeable. More
people will know about the four temperaments and their humors
when you understand this ancient art and tell them about it. I
hope you will. Here are some hints for getting others dear to you
interested in balancing their humors so their temperament will
be at its best:

If your friend or family member tends to the choleric humor,
show her how this book can lead the field in self-help and personal empowerment, so that she can see it assisting people to
become winners in their lives.

If she tends to the sanguine humor, she will be interested in
knowing how this book will be a meaningful and popular book
that speaks the truth to people about themselves and makes them
better able to communicate with others and have more fun and
adventure in their lives.

If your friend or family member tends to the melancholic
humor, she will want to hear how effective this book will be in getting people to be more productive and creative and in helping them
avoid the blind alleys and confusions of life and relationships.

And if she tends to the phlegmatic humor, she will want to find out how this book creates a new standard in its field, a book on which people can rely for help to improve their lives and relationships by giving them greater confidence and energy to do the task.

You may ask as a practical matter, what can you do when family members are all different humors? Are meals impossible to plan?

I believe this is where we got the idea of a "balanced" meal, which is so often touted as an excuse not to teach or learn about biochemical individuality and idiosyncratic nutritional needs. At least theoretically, if there is sufficient quantity and variety of healthy foods available at each meal, each family member will tend to eat the right things, assuming each person is already in healthy balance so that cravings can't get the best of them.

The main challenge for the family cook is to make sure everyone has breakfast (don't let the melancholics and phlegmatics skip it) and make sure everyone has a dinner meal at least two hours before bed (don't let the melancholics and sanguines snack late at night). Everyone does best with their main meal at lunch, but we all know how unlikely that is today for most people, when for the vast majority of people lunch is only on a short break in the middle of a day of work devoted to other people's agendas. But for those who have control of their day, or parents who are at home with small children getting them off to good eating habits, make lunch a pleasant, rich, social, nutritious event.

Another important thing to keep in mind is that refined, over-processed, and fractionated foods, whether carbohydrates or fat, are good for no one and can distort the humors of anyone. Another way you might think of these foods is to look at their color. These foods tend to be the white foods—white sugar, white flour, white breads, pasta, toasted cereals, white salt, and clear, colorless oils. These foods cause physical and emotional imbalance, creating greater stress for anyone who is trying to keep everyone in good humor around the house. What artist would want to paint a canvas with only white and clear, or compose music with only one tone and rhythm?

The simplest thing for the cook of the house to do is to minimize the availability of these foods and seldom prepare them.

The Humors in Raising Children

THIS IS MUCH too broad a subject to explore in depth here, but some hints for parents to contemplate may be helpful. First, children are fully formed temperamentally almost from the start. Their little spirits are clearer than ours as to their preferences and comfort zones. Parents would do well to respect these and honor the child's path of self-discovery. There is much you can do to keep your child on an even keel and make home life more harmonious, by applying the corrections in this chapter to your children.

It may be helpful here to outline the learning styles of children of the different temperaments, so that you can minimize friction and maximize the pleasure of learning. Melancholic dominant children who are slow to read may love to listen. They respond deeply to music and books read aloud. Reading comes easily when they know what it will sound like and can create the pictures and sounds in their heads.

Phlegmatic-dominant children want to touch everything. The phlegmatic humor is more influential in children than adults anyhow, perhaps because the pituitary hormone is more active during their physical growth periods. It follows then that children may learn best by touching things. Yet while they are in some of their fastest-growing stages, we try to tie them to desks and teach them through listening and reading words.

Sanguine children are very intuitive because of being so sensitive to senses that others often ignore. Taste and smell are deemphasized in Western culture except when it comes to fast-food advertising. Sanguines usually consider themselves gourmets more often than do other humoral types. As for learning, sanguines are often like sponges, picking up ideas that others don't pay much attention to. They look for nuances everywhere and connections and correspondences that may interest no one else.

Choleric children can be quickly bored by school. They learn reading quickly in most cases because they are visually responsive, academically competitive, and eager to explore the power dynamics on the playground, or how to duplicate the dominance that the teacher exerts.

The tremendous variation in learning styles of children is just one reason that good teachers deserve appreciation, and that schools may not be the best or most efficient way to teach all children or prepare them for life and learning. In a home education situation, a caring parent may easily adapt learning to the style of the child, or if challenged may learn to recognize the child's style and adjust lessons easily and effectively.

From the student's point of view, a mentor or teacher who is willing to explore, recognize, and nurture a child's particular gifts and humoral strengths can make all the difference. In a word, tolerance, understanding, and loving guidance will go a long way in making your family life fun and productive with the help of the four temperaments.

Focus meals instead around these two things: 1) quality, natural protein foods and 2) nonstarchy vegetables, all organically produced if possible. Supplement these with foods naturally rich in good-quality fat, like seeds, nuts, butter, and olives. Let the family eat all they want of these, since this dietary approach comes closest to the original eating patterns of humanity before we figured out how to mechanically and chemically manipulate our foods. The natural fiber, moisture, and micronutrients will help regulate the family's appetite and tastes. These help everyone stay in balance. Then urge moderation for any natural flavors they want to add and for any grain-based products or fruits they want. Encourage each family member to snack only on the foods that maintain their humors in balance.

For the rest, educate each child as early as you can about what makes them feel best, and don't let them snack on their humoral favorites. Save these for part of a "balanced" meal. In my family, as I mentioned in the Introduction, my son wanted an apple as we cooked dinner and my daughter wanted some hard cheese. Then they would bicker until supper. We just reversed the snacks and, to their amazement, the fighting stopped. Both could eat their desired foods with dinner, so no deprivation, but they each stayed "in good humor"!

Some may wonder whether it is better to adjust in one area at a time or to try to make all the changes at once. This is up to you. Actually, it really depends on your humor. Sanguines will tend to take on all changes that are indicated all at once. Phlegmatics will tend to experiment gingerly with one at a time. Do what suits you! Follow your humor. But don't give up until you get results or get an indication that you're moving in the wrong direction.

Shedding Light on Popular Controversies

I AM OFTEN asked if the humors shed any light on two popular controversies of the day, whether the high-carbohydrate diet or the low-carb diet is preferable for health or weight control, and whether meat-eaters or vegetarians do best.

There is a good deal of discussion and advocacy today about grain-based diet plans and which is healthiest, a low-carbohydrate plan or a high-carb plan. It is impossible to go into this controversy deeply here. But it is not hard to see from a study of the humors that any kind of concentrated carbohydrates will cause problems for each dominant humor, though for different reasons. The melancholics should avoid them altogether because of their tendency to blood sugar problems. But anyone can develop this condition with the high sugar content of today's popular offerings.

Meanwhile, the cholerics will tend to overeat if they mix protein and fat with carbs. The sanguines will get carried away easily with creamy, gooey spreads or fillings in carbohydrate dishes. And the phlegmatics can suffer symptoms from a cereal and milk-based diet. The tendency of particular carbohydrate sources to stimulate the pancreatic production of insulin is of course another factor to consider. The glycemic index, which helps to distinguish those foods that are easier on the balance of energy production, can be important to people of all temperaments today.

Though it has been said that every great civilization has been built on one or more indigenous grains, it should be noted that it was the poor and the laborers who lived short, hard-working lives on these grains, plus alcohol from their fermentation, while the privileged in each culture thrived on a more nourishing diet like the two-point plan above.

As for the question of vegetarianism, there are numerous reasons to avoid various kinds of animal products that we can't possibly explore now. But it can be noted that dietary investigation of healthy traditional tribal populations shows that they each have developed diets that make use of virtually anything edible in their environment, including whatever animal foods are available. No totally vegan society has been found in nature. That having been said, it is clear that some humoral temperaments must take more care than others to balance their intake of meat. Cholerics and sanguines can often do better with less, melancholics and phlegmatics with more. No one must eat red meat or hoofed animals to maintain their health and humoral balance. But all must find a good-quality source, hopefully several, of protein. If you avoid chicken and fish also, this might be challenging in today's market.

Those who eat meat must do their best to find farms whose animals are maintained in a healthy state free of medications, growth stimulants, and artificially fertilized feeds. Investigate thoroughly before you jump on the soy bandwagon. Soy meat substitutes are simply another step in the refinement of foods. Sugar and white flour cover the carbohydrate category, refined and hydrogenated oils cover the fat category, and refined soy products now offer us fractionated, overprocessed protein products. Good for profits, bad for health.

The sophisticated observation, interpretation, and application of the science and art of the humors is still evolving. As our culture and lifestyles, at work and at play, evolve, and we alter our environments outdoors and indoors, we are constantly affecting the balance of humors in each of us.

So please consider yourself a participant in the evolving understanding of the four temperaments and their underlying humors. Now, after having read nearly to the end of this book, at the very least you have developed a somewhat deeper awareness of what goes on in your mind, body, heart, and soul. At the very best, you have developed a powerful new tool to keep your body healthy, your mind serene, your heart in love, and your soul in joy.

In the next chapter you will meet eight people who are prototypical for their temperament when in harmonious balance, or good humor. As you hear their descriptions, you will have the opportunity to review all that you have absorbed from this book. Each detail of these characters can have more meaning for you than ever before and will add to your insights about people and perhaps, about yourself. Remember that few people actually resemble these folks exactly, since each person is a unique combination of the strengths and weaknesses of the four humors as well as other factors. You may, however, get a clearer awareness of how brilliantly the diversity of human character and makeup creates a community that can be fun and healthy and productive for all, as long as we respect and honor this diversity. You may come to appreciate also how profoundly we are connected to all of the natural world through earth, wind, fire, and water, and how necessary and important each of us is to the rest of the world.

☀

The progress of a disease is never faster than the speed with which it may be cured and, so long as the administration of remedies begins with the onset of the malady, recovery may be expected. But when the disease has a start because it lurks unseen within the body, a sufferer seeks treatment not when first attacked but only after his malady has gained a firm hold. *(p. 146)*

A malady flourishes and grows in its accustomed circumstances but is blunted and declines when attacked by a hostile substance. A man with the knowledge of how to produce by means of a regimen dryness and moisture, cold and heat in the human body, could cure this disease too provided that he could distinguish the right moment for the application of the remedies. He would not need to resort to purifications and magic spells. *(p. 251)*

If they knew what caused their sickness they would know how to prevent it. To know the cause of a disease and to understand the use of the various methods by which disease may be prevented amounts to the same thing in effect as being able to cure the malady. *(p. 145)*

—HIPPOCRATES (460–377 BCE), in Lloyd, *Hippocratic Writings*

CHAPTER 10

Your Personal Best:
Eight Archetypes of Good Humor and the Ultimate Chart

When the elements divide the qualities equally between themselves, health and prosperity prevail.

—ALBERTUS MAGNUS (1193–1280), *Of Effects in Nature,*
in Thorndike, *A History of Magic and Experimental Science,* p. 553

IN THIS CHAPTER, we can take one more pass at the four humoral temperaments, manifested in four male and four female characters described here. As you read about these people, imagine how you or the people you know are like them or unlike them. And think to yourself what each characteristic mentioned tells you about the humoral balance of that person. Also, imagine what kind of person each character might be attracted to for romance, as a colleague, or as a mentor. Notice how each person is confident with his or her own personal preferences but has also found a lifestyle that keeps these from turning gifts into gripes.

Remember, each of us is a combination of these archetypes. No one is less perfect than the next person because he or she is not the picture of a humor. Indeed, the most attractive, balanced, flexible person is often the hardest to identify by humor. So use these profiles to learn yet more about yourself and your relationships, and to enrich your life. After meeting these eight people, you can play with the Ultimate Chart, which will follow their profiles and end the chapter. I hope it will stimulate you to further exploration and adventure with your temperament and the four humors. The best exploration is your own observation, play, and enlightened discovery.

Charger Carl

CARL IS A large man with broad shoulders and narrow hips. Muscles seem to grow on him naturally. His jaw is square and his brow wide and straight across. His lips are thin but his smile broad. His skin is coarse and rosy. He attracts people to him wherever he goes. He loves being around people and sharing his vision of how to get things done. He likes to be in control of his own life and the situation around him. He inspires cooperation and hard work in others and never shrinks from hard work himself. He loves physical challenges of strength and endurance. He loves the outdoors, especially when it challenges him to show his stamina and power. He can go long periods without thinking about food but loves a great meal when it's time. He prefers meat and hearty soups to any dainties. He feels deep responsibility for all those dependent upon him and his leadership, and he expects others to fulfill their responsibilities as he does his. He learns quickly by intuition, and he trusts his gut feelings. He likes to see things for himself and likes to talk about hard realities but always with an eye on what must be done next. He likes light and progress in everything. He has large square hands that he puts to powerful use. His gait is strong and steady. He loves to pick a goal, make a plan, and achieve it.

Do you feel a lot like Carl or wish you were like him? Do you know people that fit this description or would, if they could only get their act together? Do people like this have a downside, or down days? What kinds of questions would engage him in conversation if you just met him?

Carl is a classic choleric gentleman at his best. Carl is at his best, balanced and inspired, but still recognizably choleric.

Jazzy Jake

JAKE HAS A sense of humor that won't quit. He is surprisingly small for the attention he can attract with his wit and all-round knowledge. He loves explaining things. He has a small mouth and face, and an early receding hair line that only makes him look more intelligent. He is romantic and not shy at all about making romantic advances. He is shapely, not tall or muscular but clearly very active and able. He likes activities that accomplish things. He likes to save effort and be efficient. He loves to see how much he can intuit in any situation, especially using his subtler senses, like smell and taste. His hands are small but toned and trained. He loves to instruct others in general knowledge and help people figure things out for themselves because this gives him so much pleasure. He loves watching children learn. His eyes are deep-set and intense. He loves meeting new people and finding out what they're all about. He likes to examine the big picture and share his insight with others. He loves to empower others to believe in themselves. He likes running and dancing and jumping, not for endurance but for the adventure of it. He likes bringing people together and wants only occasional time to himself. He'll eat almost anything, but what he likes best are creamy and crunchy things, rich seafood and vegetables in herbal or spicy sauces. He loves the tastes and smells of cooking, and loves the community and camaraderie it represents.

Do you know a Jake? Does his confidence surprise you or make you envious? Or are you a lot like Jake yourself? How would he and Carl best interact in a business partnership?

Jake is a classic sanguine gentleman. When the sanguine is in balance with the other three humors that influence his soul, he is at his best, but still recognizable as a sanguine.

Wood-Nymph Wendy

WENDY IS TALL, slender, with a soft oval face. She has a brilliant broad smile, with ample lips. Her eyes are set shallow, with entrancing lids covering her beautiful large eyes. She has sloping, smooth shoulders, delicate limbs, an hourglass shape, and ample breasts. She adores things creative and colorful. She likes to make things, and is especially ingenious and meticulous with creative projects. She loves to work intensely for an hour or two and then do something fun and spontaneous before she returns to work. Her favorite time of day is the morning, and often she likes to just sleep in and let her fantasy fly. She loves to indulge in food, trying new things, but she always returns to her favorites—fresh tasty vegetables, lean meats like shrimp, lamb, or chicken breast, and sweet fruits, like strawberries and oranges. She loves to be off by herself and is enthralled by the wonders of nature. She is romantic and loves attention, but also loves her freedom and to do things on her own terms in her own time. She loves music and is especially sensitive to people's voices and tone. When she meets new people she feels shy and waits to see if they will accept her as she is. Her enthusiasm shines once she knows you and her excitement is infectious. She wants most to enjoy life and help others do the same. She loves the creativity of children. She likes to know the rules in any situation, and she also likes to make up her own mind whether they apply to her. She likes speed and beauty, flowers and birds. She loves museums, but she also loves movement, running, dancing, and flights of fancy. She projects a strong vision of a beautiful, artistic world.

Who do you know that could be a Wendy? Are you such a woman or would like to be? Or would you just love to meet such a woman? Or would you find it hard to relate to a woman like Wendy? All answers are okay. They all depend on your own humoral tendencies, as well as on your gender.

You might want to make a list of the Wendys or potential Wendys you know. Are there some people you know that should be like Wendy but who exhibit a dark side that exaggerates their good qualities into exasperating faults?

Wendy is a classic melancholic lady. When this influence is in balance with the other three humors in Wendy's soul, she is at her best.

Faithful Amanda

AMANDA IS SLIGHT of build and youthful. No one can guess her age. She has delicate hands and feet, a youthful torso, and rounded features all round. Her face is soft and rounded too, with cute, intense eyes, a ready smile, small mouth, and expressive lips. Her cheeks are plump and light. Her forehead is rounded and smooth. Amanda loves to befriend animals and people alike. She loves to take on a task and see it through no matter how long and

Shakespeare
and the Humors

IF YOU WOULD like to explore the use of the humors in one of Shakespeare's famous comedies, here is your opportunity. Most Shakespeare readers gloss over these slightly archaic words, assuming they just add some color to Shakespearean dialogue. But the Elizabethan audiences got all the nuances, just as we can laugh twice as hard at a contemporary comedy like *Seinfeld* on TV than could someone who didn't live through the contemporaneous events and popular culture that's embedded in the language and incidents on the show.

I've underlined the words in this passage that appear to have humoral or elemental overtones, and also those words that refer to the popular debate at the time over scientific cures versus the power of divine intervention. You may be well on your way, by now, to having lots of fun with your humors and those of others, as these actors and their characters did over 400 years ago.

FROM SHAKESPEARE'S *All's Well That Ends Well*
[The play opens with banter between Helen and a male friend where he urges her that . . .]

[Virginity] 'Tis too _cold_ a companion. . . .

[The Countess questions Helen about her love for the Countess's son Bertram.]

Countess: *What's the matter,*
That this _distempered_ messenger of _wet_,
The many-colored Iris, rounds thine eye?

Helen: *I still pour in the <u>waters</u> of my love,*
And lack not to lose still. Thus, Indian-like,
Religious in mine error, I adore
The <u>sun</u>, that looks upon his worshiper
But knows of him no more.

[Helen is determined to cure the king of a dire illness and prove her worthiness to her love.]

Countess: *But think you, Helen,*
If you should tender your supposed aid,
He would receive it? <u>He and his physicians</u>
<u>Are of a mind; he, that they cannot help him,</u>
<u>They, that they cannot help</u>. How shall they credit
A poor unlearned virgin when the schools
Emboweled of their <u>doctrine</u>, have left off
The danger to itself?

[She sees the king, who resists her offer but then becomes intrigued with her confidence.]

King: *Art thou so confident?*
Helen: *The great'st Grace lending grace,*
Ere twice the horses of the sun shall bring
Their <u>fiery torcher his diurnal ring,</u>
Ere twice in murk and <u>occidental damp</u>
<u>Moist</u> Hesperus hath quenched his sleepy lamp,
. . .
<u>What is infirm from your sound parts shall fly,</u>
<u>Health shall live free, and sickness freely die</u>.

[The son Bertram, whom Helen loves, listens as two friends marvel at the king's sudden cure.]

Lafeu: *They say miracles are past, and we have our <u>philosophical per-</u>*
<u>sons</u>, to make modern and familiar, things supernatural and causeless.
. . .

To be <u>relinquished of the artists</u> [experts]—
Parolles: *So I say.*
Lafeu: *Both of <u>Galen and Paracelsus</u>—*
Parolles: *So I say.*
Lafeu: *Of all the <u>learned and authentic fellows</u>—*
Parolles: *Right. So I say.*
Lafeu: *That gave him out incurable—*
Parolles: *Why there 'tis. So say I too.*

. . .

Lafeu: <u>*A showing of a heavenly effect in an earthly actor.*</u>

[The play makes fun of the learned physicians who declared the case hopeless, while miraculous intervention has come in the form of the charming Helen.]

—William Shakespeare, *All's Well That Ends Well,* I.1.144; I.3.156–58, 209–13, 242–48; II. 1.162–71; 3.2–26, in Harrison, *Shakespeare, The Complete Works*

patiently she must work. She loves the teamwork of a project planned and executed well. She works steadily at a task, whether in play or work. She prefers light physical activity to heavy and likes light aerobics, swimming, walking, and other activities she can do casually with friends around. She likes to dress comfortably and loves to make others feel comfortable. She quickly volunteers to help others less fortunate than herself and loves a good laugh. Good cheer is a hallmark of her demeanor. She sets high value on loyalty and expects relationships to be steady and longlasting once established. She takes her time jumping into new experiences but loves to touch things to really experience them. She relates especially well to children and feels no hesitation in acting like a kid herself. Playfulness is an important part of her personality. She has energy for things she sets her mind to, but she loves to take a well-deserved rest when day is done. Late morning is a favorite, productive time. Amanda likes fruits and milk products best and doesn't think a lot about eating. She'll often choose a snack on the run. She likes cool balmy weather and sweet summer nights.

Who do you know that Amanda reminds you of? Do you feel like her at times? Would Carl be attracted to her, or she to Carl? How would she and Wendy get along? Are you thinking you may know these people? Is Amanda always bouncy and cheery? What can bring her down? I wonder.

Amanda is a classic phlegmatic lady. When the phlegmatic humor is in balance with her choleric, melancholic, and sanguine humors in her being, her soul will be happy.

I hope you can see that each of these four people are wonderfully attractive in their own right yet very different from each other. Do you think knowing each other's personal likes and dislikes might help them get along, have more fun, and be more productive together in any number of situations?

Each of them epitomizes a different one of the four classic humors. Traditionally, Wendy and Amanda represent the more feminine forces and Carl and Jake represent the more masculine forces. But there are also many people who are characterized by these humors and yet are the opposite gender. As you meet these next four, notice with your now well trained eye what they have in common with their opposite-gender counterpart and also consider how they might pair up at a social gathering, as happy life partners, fun or inspiring friends, or successful business associates.

Chairperson Donna

DONNA IS A woman's woman. She stands tall and square, strong shoulders, narrow hips, ample bosom, and proud of it. She doesn't mince words and likes to be in charge. She drives hard and expects others to do the same. She also plays hard, at golf, tennis, or competitive walking. She has a smooth, large face, wide brow, strong jaw, and broad smile. She dresses for success and exhorts people to demand more of themselves. She loves to get things done and even when she chooses to relax she often finds herself in a leadership role. She acts first on her intuition and asks questions later. She collects capable people around her and trusts the people she has picked to help her accomplish her goals. She wants her children to be ambitious and independent and tries to set a great example. She likes dinner best of all, cooks for results, eats fast, and sets a pace of tireless energy. She is compassionate toward those in need but is impatient for solutions to help get them on their feet. Sustained effort toward a worthwhile goal is her hallmark.

Have you met Donna? Can she make you feel tired? Does she run your local community group? Or are you she? Does she remind you of Carl? How would their conversation go if they met at a personal growth conference?

Donna is the female side of the choleric. Like Carl she is a driver, a natural leader, strong and decisive.

Charmer Rachel

IF YOU WANT to get a party organized, call Rachel. She loves to interact with people and offer them something neat. She is petite, with a small waist, curvy hips a little more generous than her perky bust line. Her face is small, with a petite mouth, dark deep-set eyes, and her hairline at the forehead comes to a little point in the middle. Her shoulders are small but square. She has a ready wit and loves jumping from the cosmic to the mundane in her conversation. She loves to think about and work on relationships and help others do the same. She has a gift for attracting people to share their life story with her. She likes physical activity that taxes her mind too, like dancing, diving, hiking, anything with evolving patterns. She loves to make noise, music, and rhythm, with instruments and voice. She loves evenings and gets reenergized easily at the end of the day. She doesn't eat much but loves creamy and well-seasoned foods, like exotic salads and dips for seafood. She loves to be where the action is and only occasionally seeks out time for herself outdoors with the moon and stars.

Do you identify with any of Rachel's traits? Who do you know that is like her? Would she want to hang out with Jake or with Carl? Would you mind spending some time with her?

Rachel is the female classic profile of the sanguine humor. Her male counterpart was Jake above. They are both excited by communication and relationships and are natural teachers. They cultivate good wit and erudition. When her humors are in balance, she is most happy and fulfilled.

Brave Brandon

BRANDON LOVES BEING his own person, a rugged individualist, with high ideals. He is always searching for the best way to accomplish things. The intensity of his efforts is frequently balanced by long periods of relaxation and play. He loves to have people around at specific times but wants little demanded of him and enjoys time to himself. He is tall, slender, with an oval face, shallow-set eyes, wide grin, broad teeth. His bones are small for his height. He loves quick spurts of energy and challenge, as in fast games like racquetball, squash and badminton, or baseball. He would rather compete than watch anytime. He loves color and sound. He loves to eat and to sleep. He likes lots of vegetables and hearty meals of soup and meat, but fish is a favorite too. His sloped shoulders and tapered arms, hands, legs, and feet make him look very elegant. He likes to be accepted as he is, and approaches relationships cautiously. He loves the outdoors, especially the mornings, though he also loves to sleep in. He loves freedom, and helping others achieve it. He's observant and loves sharing his observations. He loves to keep his mind active analyzing things and is surprised every time it shuts down to refuel. He is artistically creative, drawn to work and play around art, painting, sculpture, architecture, or sophisticated mental structures like astronomy, math, or computer software design.

Who among your colleagues, friends, or relatives reminds you of Brandon? Can you identify with him?

Brandon is the classic male counterpart to Wendy, our melancholic. At his best, his primary tendency toward the melancholic humor is nicely balanced by the choleric, sanguine, and phlegmatic.

There's one more profile of your eight, the male phlegmatic.

Solid Sam

EVERYONE ENJOYS SAM as a faithful friend. He loves to care about people. Loyalty counts high with him and it begins with his approach to others. He is of small and youthful build. Few can guess his age. His skin and smile have a special youthful look. He avoids strenuous exercise but loves to play with friends, swimming, softball, golf, or walking. He loves to listen to people's experiences. He likes to do any task really well, to the last detail, and loves to hear praise for a job well done. He plans his work so that it will achieve the most for the greatest number. He prefers to develop a plan rather than invent one, because he knows his strength is in his steadiness, level-headedness, and devotion to a cause. He loves to laugh and to do fun things like children do, whether going to amusement parks or playing board games or with animals. His bone structure is slight, but his size hides his impressive stamina when there's a good reason to do the work. He doesn't pay much attention to eating, preferring to put his attention on the company. He likes cheese, fruit, and snacks, and loves to help entertain others with food. He has found he does best with regular meals and good-quality meat or bean dishes, though ethically he would like to be vegetarian.

Who do you know that resembles Sam? What do you share in common with him? Does he remind you of Amanda? Would he go for Rachel or Donna, in your opinion?

Sam is of the phlegmatic humor, like Amanda, his female counterpart. His solidity and faithfulness are unmatched, as well as his youthful exuberance.

Did you recognize these folks as ideal representations of each humor? If you played the matchmaker game, would you have put Carl with Amanda, Jake with Wendy, Donna with Sam, and Rachel with Brandon? If you need a memory jog about the various humoral characteristics, these portraits can be helpful. You can also refer to the more analytical charts you have seen throughout the book and to the Ultimate Chart I am about to give you.

You now have had a bird's-eye view of the four temperaments and their humors, forward, backward, inside, and out, though still not with all the detail, color, depth, and breadth I wish I could impart. I hope you have found them intriguing, helpful, fun, and enlightening.

The Ultimate Chart

ONE OF THE most fun and intriguing things you can do with the four temperaments is to see how many different sets of four symbolic qualities you can align with the humors and elements.

As we have seen, the number four has deep roots in Western culture. Please play wildly with the correspondences I have brought together here from thirty years of playing, and add your own.

In her book *Seventy-eight Degrees of Wisdom: A Book of Tarot, Part 2: The Minor Arcana and Readings*, Rachel Pollack identifies just a few of the many suggestive fourfold correspondences that resonate through the history of Western thought. She writes,

> The number four has figured very strongly in human attempts to understand existence. Because our bodies suggest this number (front and back, right and left sides) we tend to organize our perceptions of the ever shifting world by breaking things down into fours. The view of the year as four seasons comes also from the two solstices and the two equinoxes. The zodiac contains twelve constellations, three times four. . . . We see these four represented in the Major Arcana on the cards of the World and the Wheel of Fortune as the four beasts shown in the cards' four corners. . . . The four creatures symbolize the zodiac, but they derive most directly from Ezekiel's vision in the Old Testament, later repeated in Revelation. Of all the four symbolisms the two that pertain most directly to the Minor Arcana are the four elements of medieval alchemy and the four letters of God's name in Hebrew, the tetragrammaton.

Some of these and more are aligned in this chart. Some of the lines will be a review of the various traits of the humoral and temperamental types you encountered in the questionnaire in Chapter 2 and in the diagrams in Chapters 3 and 4, or in later chapters. Others may be new to you, suggesting unexplored links to other disciplines and systems of thinking.

There are others that do not appear here at all. For example, I have not attempted to talk about color, fragrances, mineral or vitamins supplements, or the Chinese system of five instead of four elements (metal and wood appear instead of air). Please refer to the resources in the Bibliography to explore these other possibilities.

In comparing other systems of classification, it is fascinating to consider the value of cross-fertilization. Conversations I have had with experts in these parallel systems and related systems (such as

Ayurvedic and Macrobiotic) have demonstrated that the same kinds of factors—eating, daily routine, environment, and so on—are relied on in these other traditions of understanding, just as in the humoral system. The result is that if a practitioner of any of these healing philosophies were presented with a person of a certain set of traits or symptoms, the analysis might proceed quite differently, but the recommendations for how the patient should proceed to make changes in his or her life would be very much alike.

You might find it intriguing to speculate how some of these differences, the idea of three in India and the Asian subcontinent, five in China and the East, and four in the Mediterranean and the West, have impacted the relationships of these three influential cultures. With a better understanding of the four humors concept we can better appreciate our own rich esoteric history of health traditions in the West and have a richer, more conscious dialogue with the Eastern traditions of health.

In the accompanying chart of correspondences, I have made no attempt to categorize the qualities listed, as I believe, by way of final review, the more random listing may prove more provocative and stimulating for you as you peruse the list. This chart often expands the awareness of people who examine it. It can open new doors, and offer a new wealth of possibilities for you.

You are sure to find some points with which you may disagree, or that just don't seem to fit even though you know your temperament. If all of this were perfected, we would know everything and be able to fix everything! We are all sharing a journey of discovery. So please, argue, discuss, challenge, and see what new insights come up.

I hope bringing these various correspondences together will be an invitation to you to further investigation, questions, contemplation, speculation, and imagination. This way you can become part of the evolution of our understanding of the four humors and enrich your world and mine as you and your loved ones achieve your most delightful temperament and your own best health and character, so all your dreams can come true.

The Ultimate Chart
of the Temperaments

Quality	Choleric	Melancholic	Sanguine	Phlegmatic
Universal element	Fire	Earth	Air	Water
Playing Card Suit	Spade	Diamond	Heart	Club
Tarot	Scepter	Pentacle	Sword	Chalice
Qualities	Hot/dry	Cold/dry	Hot/wet	Cold/wet
Sensory focus	Eye	Ear	Nose/tongue	Hand/foot
Leadership	Commander	Sage	Wizard	Master
Preoccupation	Control	Analysis	Affinity	Loyalty
Best career track	CEO	Artist/analyst	Teacher	Social advocate
Relationship style	Competition	Competition	Cooperation	Cooperation
Dominant body/face shape	Square	Oval	Heart	Round
Metabolism	Fast	Fast	Slow	Slow
Preferred body fuel	Fats	Carbs	Fats	Carbs
Craved junk food	Salt/meat	Sugar/caffeine	Fat/spice	Milk/sugar
Stress response gland	Adrenal	Thyroid	Gonads	Pituitary
Season	Summer	Fall	Spring	Winter
Four directions	South	East	West	North
Anger symptom	Dominate	Withdraw	Argue, weep	Rebel, cry
Joy symptom	Grand vision	Creativity	Party	Play
Movie snacks	None	Chocolates	Popcorn	Milk shake
Best healthy snacks	Vegetables	Protein/fat	Vegetables	Protein/fat
Healthy diet deletions	Less meat	Less carbs	Less fat	Less milk
Healthy diet additions	More vegetables	More protein	More vegetables	More protein/ vegetables
Typical sleep patterns	5–6 hrs	Irregular, 5–10	Regular, 7 hrs	8–9 hours
Sleeplessness	Often	Occasionally	Rare	Occasionally
Alcohol preference	Hard liquor	Beer/wine	Tart, flavored	None
Weight gain	Upper body	Middle	Lower body	Equal distribution

Quality	Choleric	Melancholic	Sanguine	Phlegmatic
Good meal plan	Small breakfast	Big breakfast	Not late in evening	Regular meals
Hands	Large, square	Long, tapered	Small, short	Small, delicate
Lips	Narrow, long	Full, mobile	Petite, shaped	Pucker
Look out!	Workaholism	Booze/Smoke	Too many hats	Too obliging
Career motivation	Big results	Freedom	Cooperation	Work well done
Reasoning style	Logic/intuitive	Linear	Rationalistic	Cumulative
Teeth	Large, square	Medium, even	Medium, uneven	Large front
Forehead	Wide	High	Narrows	Big round
Esoteric gender link	Male	Female	Male	Female
Yin/yang—macrobiotic	Yang	Yin	Yang	Yin
Ayurvedic (roughly)	Pitta	Kapha	Vata	Kapha
Morphology (roughly)	Endomorph	Ectomorph	Mesomorph	Mesomorph
Libido	Steady	Wax/Wane	Often	Seldom
Favorite mealtime	Dinner	Snacks	Breakfast	None
Favorite (not best) diet	Meat	Vegetables, pasta	Shellfish	Milk, fruit
Best diet	Low calories	Low carbs	Small portions	Low milk/sugar
Weight loss	Fast	Fast	Slow	Slow
Favorite games	Competitive	Fast, varied	Intellectual	Mild, steady
Favorite sports	Tennis, golf	Squash, track	Gym, swim	Walk, bike
Perspiration	Lots	Varies	Moderate	Light
Indigestion	Rare	Often	Rare	Often
Headaches	Rare	Often	Rare	Often
Women—PMS/cramps	Rare	Bad	One day	Very little
Colds/allergies	Rare	Often	When tired	Often
Taste (Paracelsus)	Bitter	Sour	Salty	Sweet
Intellectual Attitude	Optimistic	Pessimistic	Pessimistic	Optimistic
Social Attitude	Believing	Skeptical	Believing	Skeptical
Fourfold hierarchy	Body	Mind	Spirit	Heart/soul
Reichian	Sympathetic	Parasympathetic	Sympathetic	Parasympathetic
Ancient Egyptian beast	Lion	Eagle	Ox	Man
Solar calendar	Summer Solstice	Autumnal Equinox	Spring Equinox	Winter Solstice
Medieval Gospel symbols	Matthew	John	Luke	Mark

Quality	Choleric	Melancholic	Sanguine	Phlegmatic
Pregnancy	Smooth	Rocky	Enjoyable	Uncomfortable
Five senses	Vision	Hearing	Smell/Taste	Touch
Mental orientation	Action	Feeling	Thought	Faith
Handling information	Impact assessment	Analysis	Process	Guidance
Greatest personal gift	Leadership	Creativity	Communication	Loyalty
Gift to a partner or group	Vision	Enthusiasm	Passion	Commitment
Disease tendencies	Acute	Acute	Chronic	Chronic
Attracted to	Phlegmatic	Sanguine	Melancholic	Choleric
Academic inclination	Competitive	Easily bored	Eager	Conscientious
Fuse/forgiveness	Slow/slow	Quick/slow	Quick/quick	Slow/quick
Energy in a group	Attractive	Shy/animated	Witty	Friendly
Conversation topic	Career	Project	Cosmos	Family
Jungian	Extrovert	Extrovert	Introvert	Introvert
Jungian too	Intuitive	Sensory	Intuitive	Sensory
Caffeine habits	With meals	Lots	Sometimes	Rarely
Most active time	Morning	2 hour cycles	Evening	Daytime
Learning style	Example	Analytical	Experimental	Mentor
Communication mode	Driver	Intellectual	Amiable	Accepting
Mode of comprehension	"I see"	"I know"	"I understand"	"I believe"
Mode of being	Do	Feel	Think	Believe

A Peek at the Future

LET THERE BE no exclusivity but rather an expansion of possibilities with the qualities linked by this chart with the four temperaments and their humors, the four elements and their seasons, the four corners, and the glands of metabolism.

The future of the four temperaments and the humoral way of understanding health and character now depends on you. What are the chances that the humors will come back into popular usage?

In the last twenty years there has been a significant reawakening of curiosity about ancient wisdom. As we closed the twentieth century, we had to face several key facts: that we had created the bloodiest century in history, that modern technology did not solve our problems and in fact created new ones that seem to stay just ahead of our technological fixes, and that the mystical, spiritual element in life, of the unseen, is perhaps an integral part of the whole picture and may help individuals, families, and cultures to survive and thrive. Each turn of the century has caused a reevaluation and usually results in a new interest in spirituality and the continuity of human sensibilities, as opposed to bigger is better, more is necessary, and human ingenuity is the be-all and end-all. This turn was no exception. If we are still here, what is it all for?

Even in Western scientific medicine, which is one of the most technically and scientifically advanced fields of inquiry with one of the biggest budgets in the world, many of the most educated leaders are letting us know that this is not all there is. Deepak Chopra, Michio Kushi, and others have led the intellectual arm of an across-the-board push toward more traditional modes of understanding ourselves and our world. Also, with a growing multiculturalism, each tradition is being challenged by others, and each has had cause to rethink their own and rediscover its riches.

The four humors is one of the cultural icons of the Western world of which we can be proud. We can use it to enrich the international dialogue about balance, wellness, compassion, health, and peace among peoples and the earth.

Science is coming full circle. Many quantum physicists are becoming outspoken about the fact that when you get to the heart of matter, you find only energy, and when you try to investigate that, you find only vibrational relationships. Isn't that what the humors are about, the relationships between things? There's no such thing as wet or dry, only more wet or more dry than the next thing. The ancient masters of the humors knew this. Relationships, not things, run the world.

Doctors have found innumerable things to kill enemies in the body and to manipulate bodily functions, but most doctors today will admit that they know little about how a body can prepare itself to be resistant to enemies of the microscopic kind, or how a body can maintain optimal body functions so that they won't need to be manipulated. This is where "alternative" health modalities come in, as well as spiritual systems both modern and ancient, for the maintenance and enlightenment of the entire organism, the whole being.

As a society, especially with the baby boom generation reaching its mature years, we don't want to be part of a population of stuck, cut, medicated, debilitated people who are dependent on doctors and drugs for their existence. Maintaining vibrant health is a high priority. More and more people are committing to learning and practicing whatever it takes to continue in good health and in full, flat-out living.

So there's lots of room for the humors to return, as well as lots of curiosity and energy to fuel their popularity. Today, when you feel a resonance with a certain new acquaintance or want to screen them quickly for various characteristics, you might ask, like millions of people do today, "What's your sign—your zodiac sign?" Maybe tomorrow you will ask, "What's your humor?"

Please write me at the Institute for Creative Solutions, through my publisher. Let me know how you are using the humors, what they mean to you, and what you would like most to hear more about. Meanwhile, I wish you good humor, and may the humors be with you!

Here is an old Irish Farewell Song—with wishes for balance among the four elements!

May the earth rise up to meet you,
May the wind be always at your back,
May the sun shine warm upon your face,
May the rain fall soft upon your fields,
And 'til we meet again,
May God hold you in the palm of God's hand.

Farewell.

And he who imitates the image of God will conquer the stars.

—PARACELSUS (1493–1541), *Astronomia Magna,*
in Jacobi, *Paracelsus: Selected Writings.*

SELECTED BIBLIOGRAPHY

Abravanel, Elliot D., M.D., and Elizabeth A. King. *Dr. Abravanel's Body Type Diet and Lifetime Nutrition Plan*. New York: Bantam Books, 1984.

Albala, Ken. *Eating Right in the Renaissance*. Los Angeles: University of California Press, 2002.

Atkins, Robert C. *Dr. Atkins' Vita-Nutrient Solution: Nature's Answer to Drugs*. New York: Fireside, 1998.

Bieler, Henry G., M.D. *Food Is Your Best Medicine*. New York: Vintage Books, 1965.

Chaucer, Geoffrey. *The Canterbury Tales*. R. M. Lumiansky, translator. Preface by Mark Van Doren. New York: Washington Square Press, 1954.

Cheraskin, E., M.D., D.M.D., and W. M. Ringsdorf, Jr., D.M.D., M.S., with Arline Brecher. *Psychodietetics: Food as the Key to Emotional Health*. New York: Bantam Books, 1978.

Chishti, Hakim G. M., N.D. *The Traditional Healer's Handbook: A Classic Guide to the Medicine of Avicenna*. Rochester, VT: Healing Arts Press, 1991.

Chopra, Deepak, M.D. *Perfect Health: The Complete Mind/Body Guide*. New York: Harmony Books, 1990.

Cleave, T. L., M.R.C.P. (London). *The Saccharine Disease: Conditions Caused by the Taking of Refined Carbohydrates, Such as Sugar and White Flour*. Foreword by D. P. Burkitt, M.D. Introduction by Miles H. Robinson, M.D. New Canaan, CT: Keats Publishing Co., 1974.

Clymer, R. Swinburne, M.D. *Diet: A Key to Health*. Philadelphia: Franklin Publishing Co., 1966.

_____, Rev. *The Mysteries of Osiris or Ancient Egyptian Initiation*. Quakertown, PA: The Philosophical Publishing Co., 1951.

Coulter, Catherine R. *Portraits of Homeopathic Medicines: Psychophysical Analyses of Selected Constitutional Types*. Washington, D.C.: Wehawken Book Co., 1986.

Craig, Hardin, editor. *The Complete Works of Shakespeare*. Chicago: Scott, Foresman and Co., 1961.

Crook, William G., M.D. *Help for the Hyperactive Child*. Jackson, TN: Professional Books, 1991.

D'Adamo, Peter J., N.D., with Catharine Whitney. *Eat Right for Your Type*. New York: Putnam's Sons, 1996.

Donovan, Maria Kozslik. *Astrology in the Kitchen*. New York: Doubleday, 1971.

Dossey, Larry, M.D. *Reinventing Medicine: Beyond Mind-Body to a New Era of Healing*. New York: HarperCollins, 1999.

Dutton, Richard. *Ben Jonson: To the First Folio*. Series: British and Irish Authors, Introductory Critical Studies. Cambridge: Cambridge University Press, 1983.

Eaton, S. Boyd, M.D., Marjorie Shostak, and Melvin Konner, M.D., Ph.D. *The Paleolithic Prescription: A Program of Diet and Exercise and a Design for Living*. New York: Harper & Row, 1988.

Fallon, Sally. *Nourishing Traditions: The Cookbook That Challenges Politically Correct Nutrition and the Diet Dictocrats*. Washington, D.C.: ProMotion Publishing, 1995.

Flanagan, Sabina. *Secrets of God: Writings of Hildegard of Bingen*. Boston: Shambhala, 1996.

Fukuoka, Masanobu. *The One-Straw Revolution*. Emmaus, PA: Rodale Press, 1978.

Garvy, John, Jr., N.D., D.Ac. *Yin and Yang: Two Hands Clapping*. Newtonville, MA: Wellbeing Books, 1985.

Gerber, Richard, M.D. *Vibrational Medicine for the 21st Century*. New York: Harper Collins, 2000.

Greer, Mary. *Tarot Mirrors: Reflections of Personal Meaning*. Introduction by Rachel Pollack. North Hollywood, CA: Newcastle Publishing Co., 1988.

Greer, Mary, and Rachel Pollack, editors. *New Thoughts on Tarot*. Symposium Journal. North Hollywood, CA: Newcastle Publishing Co., 1988.

Hall, Ross Hume, Ph.D. *Food for Nought: The Decline in Nutrition*. New York: Vintage Books, 1974.

Harrison, G. B., editor. *Shakespeare, The Complete Works.* New York: Harcourt, Brace & World, 1952.

Hauschka, Rudolf. *Nutrition.* Translated by Marjorie Spock and Mary T. Richards. London: Rudolf Steiner Press, 1983.

Hoff, Linda Kay. *Hamlet's Choice: Hamlet—A Reformation Allegory.* Lewiston, NY: Edwin Mellen Press, 1988.

Horgan, John. *The End of Science: Facing the Limits of Knowledge in the Twilight of the Scientific Age.* New York: Helix Books, 1996.

Howell, Edward, M.D. *Enzyme Nutrition: The Food Enzyme Concept.* Foreword by Linda Clark. Wayne, NJ: Avery Publishing Group, 1985.

Jacobi, Jolande, editor. *Paracelsus: Selected Writings.* Translated by Norbert Guerman. Foreword by C. G. Jung. Bollingen Series XXVIII. Princeton: Princeton University Press, 1979.

Jung, Carl G., editor. M. L. von Franz, Joseph L. Henderson, Jolande Jacobi, and Aniela Jaffe, *Man and His Symbols.* Introduction by C. G. Jung. New York: Dell Publishing Co., 1972.

Kadans, Joseph M., N.D., Ph.D. *Encyclopedia of Fruits, Vegetables, Nuts and Seeds for Healthful Living. With Symptomatic Locator Index.* West Nyack, NY: Parker Publishing Co., 1973.

Kroeger, Otto, and Janet M. Thuesen. *Type Talk: The 16 Personality Types That Determine How We Live, Love, and Work—Based on the Myers-Briggs Type Indicator.* New York: Dell Publishing Co., 1988.

Kushi, Michio. *The Book of Macrobiotics: The Universal Way of Health and Happiness.* Tokyo, Japan: Japan Publications, 1977.

Larsen, Robin, Ph.D., editor. *Emanuel Swedenborg: A Continuing Vision.* New York: Swedenborg Foundation, 1988.

Lloyd, G. E. R., editor. *Hippocratic Writings.* Translated by J. Chadwick and W. N. Mann. Introduction by G. E. R. Lloyd. New York: Penguin Books, 1978.

Mackenzie, Linda. *Inner Insights: The Book of Charts: Alternative Medicine & Awareness Charts.* Manhattan Beach, CA: Creative Health & Spirit, 1996.

Monte, Tom, and the Editors of *EastWest Natural Health. World Medicine: The East West Guide to Healing Your Body.* New York: Jeremy Tarcher/Perigree, 1993.

Nearing, Helen. *Simple Food for the Good Life: An Alternative Cook Book.* New York: Delacorte Press, 1980.

Newman, Barbara. *Sister of Wisdom: St. Hildegard's Theology of the Feminine.* Berkeley: University of California Press, 1987.

Page, Melvin, D.D.S. *Degeneration—Regeneration.* St. Petersburg Beach, FL: Nutritional Development, 1949, 1980.

Pernoud, Regine. *Hildegard of Bingen: Inspired Conscience of the Twelfth Century.* New York: Marlowe & Co., 1998.

Poesnecker, G. E., M. D., D. C. *The Clymer Health Clinic: It's Only Natural.* Landsale, PA: Ad Ventures, 1975.

Pollack, Rachel. *Seventy-eight Degrees of Wisdom: A Book of Tarot. Part 2: The Minor Arcana and Readings.* Hammersmith, London: Aquarian/Thorsons, 1983.

Price, Weston A., D.D.S. *Nutrition and Physical Degeneration.* New York: Paul B. Hoeber, 1938.

Reich, Wilhelm. *The Cancer Biopathy. Volume 2 of The Discovery of the Orgone.* Translated by Andrew White with Mary Higgins and Chester M. Raphael, M.D. New York: Farrar, Straus and Giroux, 1973.

_____. *The Function of Orgasm.* New York: Simon and Schuster, 1973.

Rohe, Fred. *The Complete Book of Natural Foods.* Boulder: Shambhala, 1983.

Rolfe, Randy. "Loosening the Grip of Cravings: The Four-Humor Concept of the Ancient West." *Macromuse* (August/September 1988), pp. 18–22.

_____. Research Notes, "Medieval Science in the Time of Chaucer." 1962 (Unpublished).

_____. *The Seven Secrets of Successful Parents.* Chicago: Contemporary Books, 1997.

Thorndike, Lynn. *A History of Magic and Experimental Science.* Vol. 3, "Fourteenth Century." New York: Columbia University Press, 1934.

Tintera, John W., M.D. *Hypoadrenocorticism.* Reprint with permission from *New York State Journal of Medicine* 55:13 (July 1, 1955).

Veith, Ilza, translator. *The Yellow Emperor's Classic of Internal Medicine.* Introductory Study by Ilza Veith. Berkeley: University of California Press, 1949, 1972.

Walker, N. W., D.Sci. *Raw Vegetable Juices.* Compiled by R. D. Pope, M.D. New York: Jove, 1977.

Watson, George, M.D. *Nutrition and Your Mind: The Psychochemical Response.* Foreword by W. D. Currier. New York: Bantam, 1974.

Acknowledgments

I HAVE MANY people to thank for their contributions to my life-long passion for knowledge about the four temperaments and their humors. I will mention just a few special mentors here. First I want to thank my tenth grade English teacher Marianne Riely for providing the opportunity for my discovery of the four temperaments, in 1962.

Next I am grateful to Dr. Jody Rubin Pinault, who taught a seminar entitled "Life in the Ancient Greco-Roman World," in which she laid out her own conclusions about the four humors. She urged me to continue my quest to find links between this ancient way of understanding and applications today.

I owe a great deal to Dr. Kenneth Fordham, who has been a mentor to me since 1980, and whose work for over thirty years at the Fordham-Page Clinic introduced me to important aspects of metabolism and the influence of the glands and hormones, adding a critical dimension to the link between the ancient temperaments and contemporary research into health, life balance, and metabolic and personality types.

I also want to express my thanks to Dr. Robert Jenkins, who followed in the footsteps of the visionary Dr. Swinborne Clymer, and taught me about the intricate relationship between individual constitutions and specific nutritional choices. Dr. Clymer's work in metaphysics and ancient philosophy helped me to discover the mystical aspects of the humors, especially the writings of Paracelsus and his later admirer, Carl G. Jung.

I want to acknowledge the important contributions of Helen and Scott Nearing, my great-aunt and -uncle, famous pioneers of simple living and natural health, whose lives set an example of trusting the wisdom of the body to support itself on what nature provides, with the help of hard work and persistent faith in the human spirit.

In addition, I want to thank Dr. Ross Hume Hall, nutritional biochemist, whose dedicated scientific inquiry and interest in my work kept me on my own path of inquiry. He predicted in the 1970s many of our health challenges today by looking at emerging food processing technologies and health habits.

I want to commend Dr. Michael Scanlon, OSA, professor of theology at Villanova University, where I completed my law degree in 1973 and my master of arts degree in theology in 1998. Scanlon served as a special mentor in my quest to gain a deeper understanding of the ancient mind, and in my coming around full circle to where I was in 1962, aiming to show how the ancient way of understanding the human condition has much to teach us today.

Thousands of others to whom I am grateful have enriched my life and given meaning to my quest as my students and clients in counseling sessions, seminars, workshops, and courses over the last twenty-five years.

I want to express my special appreciation and love to my husband, Jay, my son, Jason, and my daughter, Tara, for their patience and enthusiasm while I tested my theories on them in my efforts to keep them all as healthy and happy as possible. I thank also my father, physician and philosopher, and my mother, sociologist and anthropologist, who lovingly shared their worldviews with me, and took me traveling in twenty-nine countries to broaden my scope of understanding. They showed that I could do anything I set my mind to, that relationships between things help define the things themselves, that nature is wise and trustworthy, and that humanity has a mission of peace and joy.

I wish especially to thank Robert Rayevsky for his masterful drawings, which have helped so much to give life to the four temperaments in all their manifestations. And I also express my thanks to my many friends and relatives who reviewed different drafts of the book and offered their helpful comments.

I want to acknowledge all my mentors in print whom I never met, whose works are listed in the Bibliography. With their help I have harvested much knowledge and conviction about the four temperaments and their humors, which I hope will be of benefit to my readers. Of course any errors are mine.

Finally, I want to express my gratitude to my literary agent, Jeff Herman, who has encouraged me for so many years, and to my editor and publisher, Matthew Lore, whose enthusiasm and skill have helped a dream come true with this book.

Randy Rolfe, J.D., M.A., has been studying, applying, and teaching the wisdom of the temperaments for over thirty years. She has practiced law, had a family counseling practice, lectured around the country and abroad, and pursued the study of nutrition, physiology, and biochemistry. Her four previous books include *You Can Postpone Anything But Love* and *The Seven Secrets of Successful Parents*. She lives with her husband of thirty-two years in West Chester, Pennsylvania.